Having a baby creates a seismic shift in the priorities and self-image of the parents, the mother especially. Even her brain rewires to allow the integration of her most precious newcomer. So whether she likes it or not, she emerges into motherhood changed at a fundamental level.

Reading and practicing the Zen meditation techniques in *Meditation for Motherhood: Gentle Zen Meditation for Conception, Pregnancy, and Birth* can allow the tectonic plates of our lives to move without earthquake damage. The sound information about the fetus and baby, the lucid explanation of the relevance and techniques of Zen concepts, and the loving energy of Brahm's compassion will give new parents much of what they need to embrace and enjoy the event and its aftermath.

My past experience of the concepts and techniques of Zen unquestionably changed my life and I use what I learned many years ago, still, every day. We're all in the school of Life. Zen lets us wake up, and listen to the teacher inside us all.

—Dr Howard Chilton MBBS, MRCP(UK) DCH, neonatal pediatrician, Prince of Wales Hospital, Royal Hospital for Women, Sydney Children's Hospital, author of the bestseller *Baby On Board, The New Baby Book* and *Babies from Top to Bottom.*

❋

Learning Zen meditation with Brahm has really changed my outlook on life and my ability to cope with whatever it throws at me during difficult times. *Meditation for Motherhood: Gentle Zen Meditation for Conception, Pregnancy, and Birth*, far from being another stress- and guilt-inducing advice tome for pregnant women, emphasizes how much we already know, deep inside ourselves, and gives practical tools on accessing that reservoir of knowledge, compassion, and wisdom.

Brahm's vast practical experience and insight is hugely valuable to me, and I believe it will prove so to readers of this book too—whatever stage they've reached in the journey of motherhood.

—Hannah James, chief sub-editor, *Sunday Telegraph's Sunday Style* magazine

＊

An absolutely brilliant book and a must-read for anyone who will be experiencing the blessing of childbirth. Brahm has the amazing gift of being able to share with those around him the benefits of living, breathing, and experiencing the joy of the present. *Meditation for Motherhood: Gentle Zen Meditation for Conception, Pregnancy, and Birth* is the key to enjoying the space that a mother will be in during pregnancy—to not let the thoughts of past predicaments or future folly cause any interference to the beautiful place that an expectant mother should dwell in during this time.

Should you be experiencing pregnancy, then you deserve the benefit of Brahm's careful, measured, and thoughtful teachings. This book will be your lamp and its pages will illuminate the pathway ahead and ensure a peaceful pregnancy. The book is a rich tapestry of research and knowledge that Brahm has woven together as a gift to those who read it.

—Hap P Hannan, bestselling author of *Look Who's Talking*, producer of *How to Avoid a Charisma Bypass*, consultant for ABC-TV's *Strictly Speaking*, media commentator, and public speaking champion

＊

I wish to express personal gratitude for your new book. I know that having such a valuable "tool kit" will not only prove invaluable to me as I now prepare for the birth of my second child, but to women around the world experiencing any of the stages of the motherhood journey.

I particularly applaud and appreciate your book going beyond the classic three trimesters of pregnancy and birth and taking your wisdom into the crucial minutes, hours, days, and weeks following the birth—now so often referred to as the "fourth trimester". This underlines the understanding that the first three months after birth are but an extension of life in the womb for the baby.

In this book, you provide a deeply welcome, calming, and credible alternative for so many mothers who experience a rollercoaster of emotions, which ends in apprehension and confusion as a result of today's almost inevitable bombardment of conflicting advice—simply not knowing who or what to believe or trust.

Ultimately, as you perceptively say, the way through this modern morass of information is stepping back and trusting one's innate instincts. I know that the calmer and more meditative one is, the easier it becomes to tap into and trust such natural intuition. May this book bring a greater peacefulness to many during their greatest adventure.

—Elvessa Marshall, project coordinator, Cancer Institute of Australia

Gentle Zen
Meditation for
Conception,
Pregnancy, and Birth

MEDITATION

FOR

MOTHERHOOD

Yogi Brahmasamhara

with a foreword by
Dr. Margaret Gottlieb

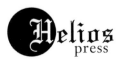

Helios
press

Helios books may be purchased in bulk at special discounts for sales promotion, corporate gifts, fund-raising, or educational purposes. Special editions can also be created to specifications. For details, contact the Special Sales Department, Skyhorse Publishing, 307 West 36th Street, 11th Floor, New York, NY 10018 or info@skyhorsepublishing.com.

Helios Press is an imprint of Skyhorse Publishing, Inc.®, a Delaware corporation.

Visit our website at www.skyhorsepublishing.com.

10 9 8 7 6 5 4 3 2 1

Library of Congress Cataloging-in-Publication Data is available on file.

Print ISBN: 978-1-63220-626-8
Ebook ISBN: 978-1-63220-750-0

Cover and internal design: Seymour Designs
Cover image: iStock
Typeset by Letterspaced
Photographs: Monde Photo
Author photograph: Pete Grayson

Printed in China

ACKNOWLEDGEMENTS
Grateful acknowledgement is made for the willing permission given by authors, researchers and scientists as well as publishers to reprint excerpts from their publications, studies and other research materials, as detailed. All effort has been made to identify, contact and acknowledge all copyright holders of excerpts from books, articles, studies and academic papers that have been quoted. The publishers would be pleased to hear from any inadvertently unacknowledged copyright holders in order to correct further editions of the book.

For all mothers everywhere, who suffer the difficulties and savour the delights of creating and nurturing new lives and bestow those tiny innocents with the ultimate gift of being able to experience their own existence. Without you all . . . we wouldn't be here.

And for Karin, just because . . .

By the same author

Half a Thousand Acres (with Dr Peter Reynolds) 1976

Awakening: A Practical Guide to Zen Meditation 2010, 2nd edition 2012

CONTENTS

PART TWO
PUTTING YOUR MEDITATION INTO PRACTICE

FOREWORD

Over many years, I have looked after a large number of intelligent, resourceful people burdened with anxiety, depression and illnesses of many different kinds. Regularly, I have discussed with them the benefits of learning meditation. Personal experience has shown me that this practice can enhance our ability to quieten the torrent of unhelpful thoughts that wear us down and, in turn, allow us to experience the richness of living more fully in the present moment. Practicing to meditate lays the foundation for self-awareness and self-mastery, taking the focus of our lives away from the not-uncommon preoccupation with fears to rediscovering the joys of the world in which we live.

In my medical practice, there was rarely enough time for me to teach patients meditation myself. My experiences recommending specific meditation classes had met with varied outcomes, some not so good, leaving me hesitant to do this. There was no obvious solution to this dilemma until two of my patients discovered a wonderful meditation class and brought this information to my attention. These classes were run by an interesting man known as Brahm, a university graduate, motor car racer and much more; a man who was now bringing his passion for teaching the life skills he learned from his own Zen meditation training to our local area.

After my previously mixed experiences I was keen to investigate for myself. To my slight annoyance, Brahm insisted that, if I was to recommend his classes, I must enroll in the whole beginners course that he ran, despite my having learned to meditate many years before. It turned out to be great wisdom in practice, as is much of what Brahm speaks and teaches. The classes were refreshingly lively, full of his personal knowledge and experience. He offered the participants the opportunity to learn a variety of techniques to help them make their own choices about how they would utilize meditation and the development of compassion as part of a range of life skills.

My patients often commented to me about the benefit to themselves and those around them that resulted from participating in Brahm's classes. New patients still do!

In his new book, Brahm has created a practical and thoughtful guide for those planning pregnancy and actual parents-to-be to use right through their pregnancy, a time of great emotional and physical change that can be both exciting and challenging. He explains the role and value of meditation to enhance harmony and wellbeing physically, mentally, and spiritually at a time when many can be plagued by worries, insecurity, and fears around their pregnancy and the impending birth.

This is the book I wish had been available when I was a scared, first-time-pregnant 28 year old, terrified of the coming birth and feeling generally ill-equipped to deal with the range of contradictory emotions forming part of my everyday mental state. I can recommend Brahm's book as a practical resource for everyone who is a parent-to-be and wanting to learn meditation and mindfulness skills that will be of value immediately and way beyond that: after the birth and really, for the rest of their lives.

DR. MARGARET GOTTLIEB
MBBS (Hons), FRACGP, DCH, MPsychMed, FACPsychMed

TO ALL WHO HELPED

Many people play a part in the long, winding journey that is the nurturing of a single-cell embryo into a fully functional little human nestled in its mother's arms. I feel similarly about the creation and writing of a book. It is never the act of just one person—the author. Without the insight and energetic encouragement of many dear people who spent precious time advising me and perusing the manuscript, as well as the wisdom and experience of medical practitioners, scholars and researchers worldwide, this book would have remained a dream.

I bow with gratitude to all the mothers-to-be and new mothers who so readily and openly shared their experiences, hopes and fears with me. I value their help in shaping the direction and contents of this book. Your honesty, sincerity and candidness rounded and smoothed the sharper edges of the thoughts and opinions I had fashioned from my own experiences and observations over the years.

I offer particular thanks to the young mothers who put pen to paper to write their own inspirational stories that are scattered through the book. It takes courage to share one of the most powerfully intimate and personal experiences a woman can have. I am humbled by their willingness to benefit others in such a loving, open way.

Very special mention must be made of Liz Seymour, a talented and thoughtful designer whose work on the cover and text is a graphic delight. My thanks also to Elvessa Marshall who, just a week before giving birth, posed so calmly for the posture photographs.

My deepest appreciation to Katie Stackhouse, my talented editor, who drew on her considerable literary and editorial wisdom when she correctly needed to harness me, while allowing me freedom of expression in such a way that I never felt restricted or inhibited in my writing. That is a rare talent . . . indeed, a shining light to others.

Rare, too, are the gifts of Pete Grayson, whose technical advice is virtually beyond peer. Hannah James is special. With warmth and humor, she worked hard to drag the author into the 21st century of social media, enabling us to spread the meditation word to a bigger world.

Dr Margaret Gottlieb has long been a friend to both the Meditation Sanctuary and me. One of the most loved and knowledgeable medical and psychology practitioners in Australia, she is not only an expert in the latest professional health practices, but has embraced meditation as a valuable tool in helping others to renew their wellbeing. She cheerfully agreed to write the Foreword to this book and the warmth of her words reflects the loving kindness that this remarkable woman offers to all.

I am a lucky man because, once more, during the gestation of this particular book, so many friends and students at the Meditation Sanctuary stood in the wings shouting encouragement. Again, special thanks for the tireless work of Beverley, Giulietta, Helen and colleague teachers Troy and Alexandra. It gladdens my heart knowing that they are always there with so much dedication and support.

Finally, my thanks to Lisa Hanrahan and Paul Dennett of Rockpool Publishing.

Again, and together, we have created a book for others. I bow humbly to you all.

INTRODUCTION

Anna came and sat quietly with me for a while after a meditation class. She was just one of many expectant mothers, sometimes joined by their partners, who come along each year to practice meditation. The story she related to me that night, through a kind of relieved smile, was astonishing.

Anna told me that, over months of practice, she had gradually increased the time she meditated every day from a few minutes to an hour. After one very peaceful practice session the previous week, she noticed that her baby had become very still. All the little kicks, the elbowing for room and swimming around just completely ceased. She didn't think much of it at first but, after three days, she became worried and made an urgent appointment with her doctor. After a thorough examination she was told that she and her baby were just fine. Her doctor smiled and said, 'He's just meditating, too!'

Several months later, Anna called me to report that everything had gone well. She was thrilled and amazed at how calm, quiet and happy her new little one seemed to be. It was at that pleasing moment that I began to realize that there just may be a correlation between a mother's level of calmness during pregnancy and delivery and her baby's emotional wellbeing.

Vanessa's call a year or so later proved just as surprising as Anna's story. Vanessa was a popular Pilates teacher and had decided to add meditation to her skills. She, too, increased the time she gave to daily practice when she became pregnant and, with her yoga background, became quite masterful. She phoned to say how thankful she was to have had her meditation mind with her during delivery. It had worked so well that she had actually fallen into peaceful little sleeps between contractions. Vanessa also reported that her little one was a delightfully calm baby.

That birth story, for me, was eye-opening. The message was that she had experienced little sense of distress or apprehension in giving birth—in fact, quite the reverse—directly attributing her calmness to meditation.

And so, the glimmer of an idea originated as I began to realize that the practice of authentic meditation may go well beyond a correlation between a calm mother and, in due course, a calm baby. I began to divine that genuine meditation could be a dynamic support resource enabling women to enjoy their pregnancy with much less anxiety, experience delivery in a far more positive manner, and have considerably fewer post-natal difficulties.

I then began to contact other new mothers who had practiced meditation at the Sanctuary before or during pregnancy and motherhood. Of the 30 new mothers I spoke to or from whom I received letters (some of which are included in this book), 26 reported a completely natural childbirth with no medical or relieving intervention at all. Of the remaining four women, one chose an epidural, one was induced (gaining relief from nitrous oxide gas), and two had cesareans (one planned because of difficulties with a previous birth and one a last-minute necessity). So, of this admittedly tiny sample of new mothers, only about 13 percent had interventions of one kind or another.

Through further research, I have since come to understand that, in the general population, more than 30 percent of pregnant women have cesarean sections either by choice or for clinical reasons (a 74 percent increase in the last 20 years). Another third of women have had an epidural, and if inductions, painkillers and augmentation are included, only 10 percent of women experience a totally natural childbirth.

(It must be noted that many interventions are the result of a mother's absolute right—and need—to relief or assistance. Moreover, while highly qualified medical practitioners have reviewed the meditative techniques and exercises discussed within this book, they are not designed to replace medical needs or interventions if or when they are required.)

Of course, my survey cannot in any way be regarded as statistically meaningful or scientifically correct. But centuries of wisdom confirm the beneficial effects of meditation on conception, pregnancy and childbirth. Listening to the many stories from meditating moms-to-be and new mothers confirmed my growing understanding that meditation can be of particular benefit to women throughout their motherhood journey.

Worldwide professional wisdom is now also gratefully and rapidly drawing meditation into the medical mainstream, understanding that a woman's emotional wellbeing, her physical health and stress levels can have a dramatic effect on her fertility, pregnancy and delivery—as well as on the baby.

Meditation for Motherhood brings together meditation and motherhood in a comprehensive, clear and logical manner. It was written to help you rediscover your own natural ability for deep calmness, to cultivate an awareness of your own needs, to discern and embrace your own inner wisdom when confronted with difficulties and to develop the patience to listen to yourself as well as your baby.

The book provides practical, step-by-step guidance on authentic Zen meditation—the most powerful, absolutely natural and deeply beneficial practice available to a woman in each of the various phases of creating and nurturing new life. It is offered in the experienced knowledge that meditation is perfectly natural (small children practice it innately) and, as a minimum, can do no harm.

But, beyond the practice of meditation and acceptance of medical wisdom, the caring mothers to whom I spoke also emphasized that the qualities of common sense, unquestionable cherishing and inextinguishable love were the main forces that carried them through the 'rough patches.' The meditation guidance in this book and certainly any advice and opinions have been specifically shaped by the naturalness of these innate mother-qualities.

I accept and promote the ancient and now prevalent wisdom that, above all, baby knows best 'what is going on.' She is the one who, from conception, has built-in expertise on knowing when and how to grow, the right time for each sense and organ to develop and how to prepare for her birth. Then, all by herself, she makes the decision to leave her first home when she is ready to go face the big wide world. Upon arrival, of course, she is acutely aware of her needs in order to survive and then, in no uncertain terms, lets you know. The parents' task is to learn how to listen to that inbuilt wisdom. Meditation is perhaps the best 'learning to listen' practice available.

I wish you well on your journey with meditation and hope that your practice of it will enhance your ever-wondrous, ever-expanding experience of motherhood—for the rest of your life.

HOW TO USE THIS BOOK

Meditation for Motherhood is divided into two parts for ready reference at all stages of your motherhood journey.

Part One introduces Zen meditation and underlines the proven benefits of practicing. It is also your textbook. This segment provides in-depth, step-by-step guidance in all the relevant meditative exercises and practices that will be of benefit to you during the different stages of conception, pregnancy, delivery and early motherhood.

For this part, I have selected for you all the classic, original and wonderful practices of Zen meditation that can be of very specific benefit on your motherhood journey. They all simply involve relearning how to become calm, poised, deeply focused, peaceful of being, awake and wiser in all the situations you may face.

You will practice the ancient art of permanently de-stressing by learning how to let go tension, right breathing, damping down the mind babble, deeply focusing on 'just this' and then dwelling within quietness. Above all, you will practice and acquire the ability to take it with you (the practice of mindfulness) as a complete support resource on your journey.

Part Two discusses how to actually apply your meditation so it is of real value to you throughout the various stages of motherhood. It looks briefly at the medical and scientific evidence of the negative role played by plain old stress and the proven benefits of using meditation to 'de-stress.' In this context, it discusses the use of health and meditation practices for couples making the effort to become pregnant, for women who may be having difficulties in becoming pregnant or who may be undergoing IVF treatment.

The most important chapters then look at applying your meditation in the three trimesters of pregnancy along with the changes both you and your baby experience as she grows and then of course, during that great event, delivery. Finally there are some words of wisdom from experts on some of the issues that mothers may face with bonding, post-natal depression, feeding, sleeping and soothing.

Meditation is deeply pleasurable, but it does require some dedicated time and effort every single day. Soon though, you will find that the time expended is a small and enjoyable price for the benefits that ripple through the rest of your life—and your baby's.

To make *Meditation for Motherhood* a genuinely helpful reference book, I recommend that you read it completely through once before commencing any exercises. This will give you a much greater understanding of the breadth of benefits available through meditation and will help you to plan your daily practice regimen.

Having read the book through, return to Part Two and bookmark the week of your pregnancy (for example, mark Weeks 7–8). Read through the commentary on those weeks again and note which exercises the Meditation Guidance Panel recommends you should now be doing. Find and bookmark those exercises in Part One and do them as recommended. It then becomes easy to follow. Just move your bookmarks forward every couple of weeks as your pregnancy progresses, practicing the relevant exercises as you go along.

It is important that you practice the exercises in the order I suggest for the very simple reason that each is dependent upon you becoming adept with the previous one. Please don't be tempted to think, 'Oh, this exercise is too easy. I shall just skip it and move on.' All the exercises have purpose and meaning and have been created and practiced over centuries . . . because they work!

As there are many exercises and skills for you to practice over the coming months of your pregnancy, I suggest that you keep a record of your progress—the date, the exercise you are working on and the time that you are spending on each one. This is an efficient way of keeping track of your progress and practice and shows you where to resume each day. You can also record your mantras and any visualizations you find helpful. This can become a lovely record of your pregnancy.

Start meditation at any time of your pregnancy

Some moms-in-the-making will have found this book either before endevoring to conceive or early in their pregnancy and they will therefore be able to maximize the potential benefits of meditation. However, others may have begun reading it later in their journey towards motherhood, some perhaps even in the weeks just before birth. Not to worry. Even if you become familiar with just the basic elements of meditation and you practice those each day, meditation will be of value to you throughout your pregnancy and delivery. No matter when you begin your practice, it will be of benefit to your wellbeing now and for the rest of your life.

If you are further into your pregnancy, I suggest you add at least 10 minutes to all recommended times, but don't overdo your practice to 'catch up'. Practice every day, focusing on the really core, unable-to-do-without elements of meditation first, such as:

* a tension-free body, right and dynamic breathing, quieting the mind techniques
* letting go techniques, open-eye meditation
* visualization, mindfulness.

Partners on the journey too

Importantly, this book is not only for moms-to-be and new mothers. The entire journey can be pleasurably enhanced if the father of the baby understands what his partner is actually doing when she meditates and why she has chosen to practice. Joining her in practicing can help him appreciate what she is doing, be more perceptive of both the mother's and the baby's needs and, of course, experience some rather exceptional benefits for himself.

Gender use in the book

As about half of my readers will have a girl and the rest will have a boy, I am faced with an interesting problem—how to refer to your baby without using the very impersonal 'it' or even 'they' (especially as bringing a new life into the world is just about the most beautifully personal experience that parents are likely to share). Swapping from 'he' to 'she' in every chapter, however, can sometimes seem to be a feverish effort to be inclusive. So, apropos of no reason at all (and as you may have already noticed), I have settled on the female gender throughout when talking about a new life.

As the significant majority of partners of pregnant women are men, I have used the male gender when referring to a partner. I am also aware that there are child-blessed, same-sex couples, one of whom may be the birth-mother and the other, the support partner. If that is you, understand that I encompass all of you equally when I use the word *partner*. I am equally aware that some moms-to-be don't have a formal partner but are supported by a friend who I refer to as a *birth-friend*. For me, *partner* and *birth-friend* are big words that cover all the good people who support our moms-to-be and new moms with love and care.

So, time now to set out on your meditation journey. Just know that if you really dare to take meditation into the lives of you and your baby, it can only have a radiant effect on you both. As I always say to my students: hasten slowly, travel well.

'I have learned that to be a mother is to give for the sole pleasure of giving. You are slowly making me a mother and I love you for it and I will always love you.'

– Barbara Martino, writing a letter to her baby in the womb, Paris 2010*

* Barbara is the woman (along with her husband Manu Bacon, and baby) featured throughout her pregnancy and delivery in the brilliant *Odyssey of Life* series by VEA. (See Recommended reading and viewing, page 242)

PRELUDE

Throughout the book are several 'little stories of encouragement' from women who practiced meditation during their maternity and who have kindly shared their experiences. I have decided to use this particular story, written by one of my dear students, Vanessa, as the Prelude for *Meditation for Mothers*. I have placed it right here because I think that the intimately personal, caring and wise way she shares the details of her meditation and motherhood journey in her own words possibly does more to encourage and enlighten moms-in-trying, moms-to-be and new mothers than the rest of the entire book. Let Vanessa's story be a light shining the way for you on your journey.

Vanessa's story

A meditative journey into motherhood

I sought out meditation in my early 30s after years of thinking that my chronic anxiety and inability to slow down was simply part of my personality—something to be endured by my family and me. I had experienced many physical manifestations of my rattling, uncontrollable mind and all of the stress that comes along with it—heart palpitations, fully fledged anxiety attacks, fear and paralysis when speaking to a room full of people (unfortunately a part of my job) and even a peptic ulcer at the ripe old age of 15.

By my 30s, I was engaged to a man I knew I loved very much. I was nonetheless suffering from mild depression and a disengagement from life. I truly believed that other people were happier, more successful and more fortunate than I. I thought this was an irrefutable fact and that it would always be this way. I would simply endure life and my future husband's role was to endure me! Despite having wonderful friends, I also worried that they would eventually see inside to the real, sad 'me' and abandon me in preference for shinier, happier people.

Finding Brahm and the Meditation Sanctuary seven years ago was life changing. I started in winter and no matter how cold or wet the night, or how strong my desire to sleep on the couch after a long day at work, I would look forward to entering that simple space. It was nothing fancy—a simple meditation hall—but it was always lovingly prepared by Brahm's helpers, who adorned the space with candles, home-grown flowers and incense.

There are two activities we did as beginners with Brahm at that time that really stuck in my mind and gave me the insight to how powerful the mind can be. The activities showed me how I could start to learn to manage my destructive, depressive and self-loathing thoughts.

As part of the first exercise, Brahm asked us to spend 10 minutes writing down all the thoughts that flitted through our minds. They could be about the sound of the rain outside the door, the smell of the candles in the room, thoughts about the other meditators sitting around us, our day at work, some unforgiven act from our childhood—anything. I am a relatively verbose person who loves to write so my page was quickly filled!

Next we were asked to go through the list putting a single line under any thought that related to the past, a double line under any thought about the future and a circle around thoughts relating to the present. Invariably, Brahm explained, examining our writing leads to a sorry conclusion. As poor, stressed-out humans we spend more than 90 percent of our precious time mulling over past events. This is useless as we can't change them! Or we fret about what is to come, which is also useless as we can't control it! So little of our attention is spent in the present—the only time that we can exercise full power and perfect perception and the only space in which change is possible.

Looking down at my list, my result was even more extreme—fragments of my burned-out mind were stuck somewhere in events from five, 10 or even 20 years ago. I realized what a mental and physical burden this was, and I felt love and compassion towards myself for having carried this burden almost unwittingly for so long. This was probably my first self-loving thought in a decade, and I wondered what wonderful things I could achieve if I could free up my mind even just a little, and how much better life would feel if I could engage more fully in the present.

The second exercise was about the mind–body connection and the power of focus. We were asked to meditate for just five short minutes to still our minds. I found it relatively easy to sink into the silence of the space of the Meditation Sanctuary and follow my own breathing, feel my ribs expand and retract and will the chaos from my mind. Suddenly, Brahm called my name, 'Vanessa!' I opened my eyes. He was looking directly at me and in the same moment a tennis ball came flying through the air towards me. With no time to think, my left hand lifted from my lap and I caught the ball.

None of this may sound remarkable, but I had the distinct feeling of my body operating of its own accord. There was no internal rattle in my head: 'Why did he yell? Why does he have a ball? Why is he throwing it at me?' I didn't have time to think. My hand just knew to lift up. I will never forget how well I caught the ball. I am right-handed and not good at ball sports but had caught it with my left hand with the precision of a baseball player almost before I was aware of what I was doing. By using such a simple example, Brahm showed me, and indeed all the other students, how powerful and intuitive a being I really was—how we really are—if we are focused. He called that experience 'satori': perfect awakeness or mindfulness.

Shortly after starting my meditation, I became pregnant. I remember the warm hug from Brahm and the genuine joy he felt for me. My belly grew and grew and I never stopped meditating—on the floor in the normal cross-legged position for as long as I could and then leaning against a chair towards the end of the pregnancy. I had opted for a natural birth, if my body and baby would allow it, and was signed up at the Camperdown Natural Birth Centre in Sydney.

I loved the idea of birthing in water and this was my goal. I knew I would need incredible focus and resilience and I was so grateful for everything I had learned in meditation in the previous months—how to control my breathing, how to still my mind, how to go inside and use positive visualization. My midwives told me that I would need to be able to relax into the birth, to open my body and let the baby travel through me into the world. Of course, there were moments of apprehension but, rather than feeling scared, it felt like a sacred duty to be performed and I felt blessed to be given this opportunity.

I often thought about the tennis ball experience and reminded myself that the calmer and clearer my mind, the more effectively and intuitively my body would work during labor. So I created an internal place for myself that I would visit in my meditations. Despite it being extremely personal, let me share it with you.

It was a place of incredible peace and beauty, a place only my baby and I inhabited. It was a subterranean cave with a shaft of light coming down like a column hitting the opal-colored water of a small, underground spring. In this space, I would be seated on a rock by the water. I saw myself pregnant and would speak to my unborn baby. I would tell her all the things we were going to do together in the birth—I would open and then push, and she should not be scared and would descend. Sometimes I pictured myself in the water—under the water—holding out my arms and seeing my baby swim into my arms.

I meditated on this incredible image over and over again, almost daily. When the time came to give birth, I found myself in the bath as planned. I had a long labor and the sensation of the contractions was entirely new. I was in the bath for approximately three hours, in the dark, with my aunt (a midwife) and my husband. We were silent—I just needed to know that they were there. For the first half of the labor I was mentally in my cave. That familiar image was so reassuring and it kept me in a state of calm and peace—so calm and peaceful, in fact, that I actually fell asleep between contractions several times.

My husband and aunt still recall how incredibly quiet I was. Then, when the contractions built and came faster, suddenly I added a new mental image on which to focus. I saw myself climbing a mountain with my unborn baby cheering me on. My aunt remembers seeing me, eyes closed, 'stepping' my feet during each contraction. Again, I did all of this silently.

Of course, all births come to a more active stage. When Saskia crowned, I suddenly felt the urge to get out of the bath and re-enter the present. She arrived into the world not much later.

Meditation helped me go into a completely unknown situation with solid ground under my feet. I knew I was strong, focused and that I would have the mental and physical stamina to bring a baby safely into the world. My daughter is now almost six years old and I know our bond today has more than just a little to do with the long time I spent with her in our 'cave', making a loving commitment to each other before she was even born.

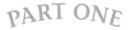

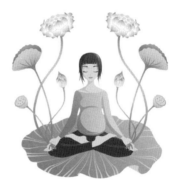

ZEN MEDITATION: PREPARING AND PRACTICES

CHAPTER ONE

Introducing Zen meditation

There are many misconceptions and myths about meditation. I was extremely blessed in my life to have met, studied and practiced with two great masters who were eminently perceptive and wise. Both of them, an Indian yogi and a Japanese Zen monk, were able to set aside the oft-associated religious and dogmatic nonsense and pass on the truth that Zen meditation is ultimately about the very way you live your life.

In a fuller sense we can also say that meditation is a journey or a path of reawakening, revitalizing and renewing our true self. This is the original, lovely self that tends to get swamped by the drudgery of leading a 'normal' life without an inner calmness or sense of joy or wonderment.

Practicing Zen meditation also enables us to reach back into our natural kindness, compassion and love until we actually become those natural qualities . . . and just simply live them. The Zen masters suggest that the 'end point' of meditation (some call it 'enlightenment') is simply turning back to your immediate dear ones and wider community but filled with loving kindness for all, the whole time . . . because you can't help it.

To the person grinding out a daily living or doubled over with morning sickness, however, that lovely-sounding journey can seem like an irrelevant ideal that is reserved for a spiritual few tucked away in a monastery or blissed-out on a misty mountain somewhere. That's why I tell my students to forget just about everything they may have heard about meditation. Instead, I tell them that meditation is the gentle, simple, utterly natural practice of getting back or renewing all the profound and perceptive skills that we had in abundance as a child.

You will understand what I mean more fully when you hold your tiny one in your arms. She will be born with pure, nature-given, meditative qualities that we adults have usually long forgotten or covered over. You will see, as she begins to adapt to her outside world, that she has a pure capacity for focused calmness, curiosity, playfulness and an instinctive ability to express joy at simple things. She will have a deep awareness of each moment of her life, totally present in her existence . . . a meditative being in the truest sense.

I often say that 'all little children are like Zen monks . . . they are our teachers'. We just have to watch, listen and learn.

The encouraging truth is that our original capacity for delighting in our existence moment by moment is still there, deep within like a beautiful, peaceful garden, just waiting to be visited again. Meditation is a powerful way of enabling us to reach back into that garden—into experiencing life with the same freedom, naturalness and attentive wakefulness of a small child. Meditation won't take away all the problems or inconveniences that continue to crop up, but if we dare to practice it until it is our natural way of living again, we can rediscover all those beautiful qualities.

Of course, along the extraordinary motherhood path, the important thing to you (and what this book is essentially about) is that meditation also offers practical, very real, positive benefits every step of the way, from conception, through pregnancy, birth and bonding. Before we work on applying meditation to genuinely enhance each of these aspects of becoming a mother (and after you've read the book through), we need now to get into preparing for it and then the gentle art of practicing it.

If you dare to take meditation into your life, you will find it is like 'getting your whole life back,' as one student said. Little by little, it will seem like the sun shining in your kitchen window on a winter's morning.

CHAPTER TWO

Preparing for meditation

Meditation is the greatest gift you can give yourself.

– SOGYAL RINPOCHE

Your first priority is to set up a meditation space of your own at home. Find a quiet place indoors where you can retreat without interruption and place some soft, flat cushions on a yoga mat or similar on the floor. If possible, choose somewhere they can be left in place so that the area becomes a little haven for quiet time each day. Later, you may find wonderful peace meditating in your garden or at a park.

If it makes you feel more at home, particularly in the early stages, adorn your meditation sanctuary with special or treasured pieces. Arranging flowers and polished river stones can make your sanctuary comfortingly personal. Sweet aromas are therapeutically calming. You may choose to light a stick of incense or, if you have breathing problems, try a little bowl of scented oil.

You might also like to have some meditation music that creates a gentle mood. There are many beautiful CDs of monks chanting, the sound of waves on the shore, the whispering of a Japanese shakuhachi flute or even the sweet sound of Tibetan bowls being played that can create an ideal background of white noise. Very soon, your special place will feel quite welcoming as you associate it with increasingly pleasant experiences.

There is no special outfit or uniform needed for meditation. Whatever loose clothes that feel comfortable as baby grows are just fine. In winter, don't wear layers of jumpers and coats but wrap yourself warmly in a shawl or robe. Beanies are good for head warmth.

Getting the most out of your meditation

It is best that you are not overtired when you practice because, if you are, you will almost certainly fall asleep. If you do, that's fine. Your body is just telling you that you need more rest and meditation is probably the very best, non-drug cure for insomnia available. Over time, however, you should actually find that practicing meditation gives you more energy.

Avoid stimulants such as coffee or strong tea before practicing or even altogether. They will make your mind excited and your body tense—the enemies of quietness. Similarly, physical exercise is a stimulant that can give you a feel-good high (which is why it is recommended for people suffering anxiety and depression). It is best then to leave your body work until after meditation.

Whether you eat before practicing depends on the length of your meditation. For a longer meditation, you should not be starving because you will be distracted by hunger. It is best not to have a large meal just before meditating either, as that draws down the energy supply for digestion, which can make you tired. I suggest a light meal only or a piece of fruit (banana is good) or a slice of wholegrain toast.

Prescription medication

I am often asked if prescription drugs such as antidepressants or blood pressure medication will affect meditation. I recommend that you never suddenly stop medication that has been prescribed wisely by a trusted medical practitioner. Some drugs taken for depression and anxiety will slightly dull the experience of meditation, but they won't nullify its value. I advise people to work sensibly with their doctors to reduce their prescription drug intake progressively, particularly antidepressants, as meditation begins to replace the work done by the drugs. In this way, countless people have become naturally drug-free over time on their way to renewed wellbeing.

Finding time to meditate

Finding time to meditate is an oft-raised issue. You will need to create time to practice because, very simply, without practice, there are no benefits. Mostly, it's just a matter of simple discipline—saving time by wasting less time or rising a little earlier. A suggestion from my Zen master was the simple principle of 'wake up, get up'. It can be difficult at first, but you soon welcome the extra time spent doing something wonderfully positive.

You can meditate any time, day or night. Many people prefer the early morning because it sets the tone for the rest of their day. I have always preferred the early morning, starting before dawn and enjoying the sunrise, the most deeply peaceful time of the day. Others prefer to come down from another busy day by practicing in the evening. This can be beneficial too, particularly if you are having trouble sleeping. Just try different times of the day until you feel you have it right.

In the Meditation Guidance Panels in Part Two, I suggest the length of time you might allocate for each session. You will find that the time suggested gradually increases up to about an hour a day as you near the time of delivery. This longer time may be broken up into two half-hour spells or even three 20-minute sessions. It is your practice, however, so you can allocate as much or as little time as you wish—as long as you do it!

Daily practice essential

It is of little value dabbling your toe in the meditative practice pond to see if it works for you or to see if you like it. You need to develop a discipline to give true and daily attention to your practice. I repeat endlessly to my students, 'no practice, no benefits'. However, when you develop 'just sitting' as a habit, the gradually developing benefits will encourage you to make practicing a most valued part of your daily life.

Difficulties with practice—time for self-kindness

Practicing meditation is not always a smooth path. At some points along the journey you are certain to become diverted by mental ruts or lost in everyday activities. When we find the journey hard going, our conditioned tendency is to allow feelings of failure to arise. But the moments of falling off the path are natural and normal. The absolute key to dealing with troubles on the journey is not to chastise yourself. Know that everyone has slipped back in their practice at some time.

If you find your daily practice becoming difficult or a chore, simply go back to an easier exercise. Even go back to the beginning. Rebuild your confidence and enthusiasm by practicing it again until you feel you have mastered it once more and then gently move on. One student experiencing difficulties told me that, 'for a while it wasn't working, but I celebrated my just sitting down and trying every, single day—and then one day it was beautiful again.'

Apprehension about starting

Having feelings of doubt at the beginning of anything new is totally natural. If you feel a little apprehensive, be reassured that all students who genuinely practice soon find that meditation is the gentlest of ways to let go all the woes, worries and disquiet, all the natural barriers to calmness and inner peacefulness.

One student said to me, 'I am happily stuck with this for the rest of my life!' How beautiful. Be encouraged. Create some time and get going on this amazing journey. It can only be of benefit to the wellbeing of you and your baby.

Understanding the concept of 'letting go'

Meditation is ultimately the practice of letting go so that we can uncover our beautiful naturalness once more. Throughout your practice, understanding the concept of letting go is intrinsic to what I call the Three Essences (which will be discussed further in chapters 4 to 6).

Briefly, however, I am not going to teach you how to relax. We are going to practice letting go tension (the First Essence). I am not going to teach you fancy yogic breathing techniques. We will practice letting go our bad habits of breathing so that we can breathe naturally and freely (the Second Essence) as we all could as a baby. Finally, we are not going to learn how to quieten our mind. We will practice letting go the babble of our thoughts (the Third Essence).

Letting go expectation before you start

Many students come to the Meditation Sanctuary full of wide-eyed expectation. Some mothers-in-waiting come along with a bubbling undercurrent of excitement, perhaps believing that learning meditation will lead to a trouble-free run to the finish line—holding the perfect babe in their arms. It may well do, but any results through the practice of meditation can only happen (or naturally come back to us) if we totally let go the expectation of a result. Starting off with high expectations only creates a barrier to the effectiveness of your practice.

My dear Japanese master, Suni Kaisan, used to say, 'I am not interested in results. I am interested in your effort. Out of your effort, the results will come.' Total wisdom. Simply sink into the calming pleasure of practicing just for the sake of practicing so the lovely skills that you reacquire will become the end in themselves, not the means to an end.

The great yogic secret is to have patience. Give undivided attention to each single step with no thought of the next. Practicing without expectation makes each moment an experience of calmness and, perhaps, even joy.

CHAPTER THREE

Comfortable postures for your practice

There is no perfectly correct way to lie down, sit or position your hands for meditation. There are, however, a number of classic Zen meditation postures that are used because centuries of practice have shown them to be balanced and comfortable, even in longer practices. You may well find your own variations to the postures in this book. That is just fine as long as you never strain or tense any part of your body in order to maintain a particular position.

Moving when uncomfortable

Until you are practiced in your preferred postures, you may find that your back occasionally hurts or your legs become stiff, sore or tingly. Various other areas of your body may also complain simply because they are not familiar with their new task. This is quite normal in the earlier days of your meditation.

There are some teachers of meditation who instruct students who experience pain or discomfort to simply suffer through it because, they say, it gives you a point of focus during practice. Ignore them totally, whether pregnant or not.

The truth is, pain is your body-friend. It is designed to let you know that something is amiss and it wants you to do something to alleviate the physical stress it is suffering. Do not ignore your body—listen to it carefully. I tell all students that if they need to move because of pain or discomfort, then they should move. But the yogic secret is when you need to move, do so, but very, very slowly and gracefully, like a ballet dancer so you 'don't spill the calm'.

For example, if you have pain in your back, perhaps twist a little to one side and then the other—but slowly. Hold any new position for a little while before moving again and you will almost certainly get relief. If your legs start protesting, either open the posture a little (by moving both legs a little further in front of you), or stretch one or both legs straight out ever so slowly while keeping your mind on your practice. If pain continues after you have moved, change the posture altogether and start again (see alternatives below). Above all, do not suffer pain or distress. Just move.

There will be times in your pregnant life when the last thing you want to do is get on the floor and meditate—especially with morning sickness. Be reassured, however, that all exercises can be done while lying down—in bed if necessary—and that keeping up your meditative practice can be hugely beneficial.

Ideal lying down, sitting and hand positions

The lying-down posture (*savasana*)

We lie down in the earlier exercises, as this is the easiest of the genuine yoga postures and perfect for easing into your practice. The right way to lie down is the first posture of *hatha* (physical) yoga—called *savasana*.

In Photo 1, you can see that the student is on her back with no part of her body touching any other part. Her arms are slightly away from her body and her ankles are a little apart. Her head is straight with eyes closed and, most importantly, the palms of her hands are face down (this is a natural posture). Place a cushion or two under your head if it makes you more comfortable.

If you are more than two or three months pregnant when you start meditating, you may find it better

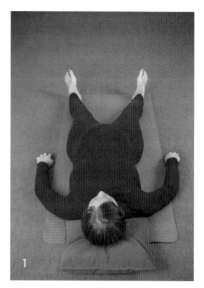

to use one of the sitting postures below, many of which you can do quite comfortably until late in your term.

Sitting posture – the Zen variation (*sukhasana*)

The Zen variation of the sitting posture is a softer version of the

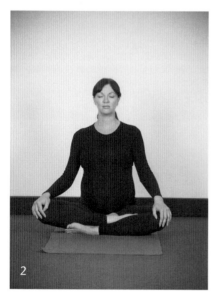

classic, yoga lotus posture and is the most common sitting posture used by Zen masters (see Photo 2). Called *sukhasana*, this is the simplest, most comfortable and balanced sitting posture.

To adopt this posture, cross your legs in a loose way so that one doesn't place pressure on the other. Experiment a little to find the best position. The back is neither rigid nor bent forward, but just comfortably and slightly arched, and never rigidly straight (too much tension). The key to this balanced posture is the position of your head. Again, experiment until you find the balance point for your head so that holding it in position requires minimal tension in your neck muscles.

If you began your meditation practice early in your pregnancy and all is well, there is virtually no reason why you can't use this posture throughout your pregnancy.

Wall posture

If any posture becomes too hard to hold, try sitting against a wall. The first wall posture is simply sitting against a wall with your legs straight out ahead of you with cushions placed between the wall and your back as well as underneath you. Many find this posture perfect for later pregnancy (see Photo 3).

If you are uncomfortable, you can raise your tail higher off the ground with two or three thicker cushions. Your legs are still gently crossed but your knees point down a little more towards the floor (see Photo 4).

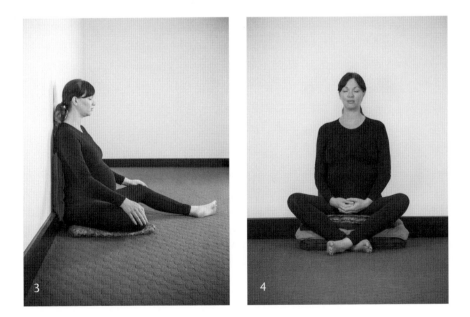

Alternatives to sitting on the floor

You may find it difficult to adopt any sitting posture on the floor, particularly when you have a large 'baby bump'. Therefore, sitting on a chair is perfectly fine for all the exercises in this book. Choose a chair that, while you are sitting on a cushion, enables your feet to be flat on the floor with your thighs horizontal to them. If the chair is a little too high, place cushions under your feet so that your legs are in a comfortable position.

Alternatively, you can sit on a lounge chair and place your arms along its armrests (if it has them) and your feet flat on the floor.

Lying on your side in later pregnancy

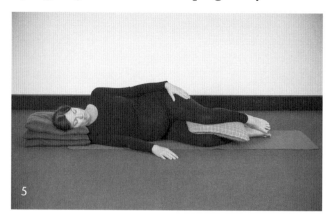

Lying on your side is another perfect posture for alleviating discomfort that may come with a big belly later in your pregnancy (see Photo 5). You may, of course, change the precise details of the posture on a daily basis according to your needs, but you can do all the exercises and meditate perfectly well while lying on your side.

Again, place a cushion or two under your head and others between your thighs and knees. You can rest the lower arm, palm down, along the mat and the other downwards along the top of your body. Both arms are then in a position that retains no tension at all.

Hand postures

The way we rest our hands while meditating is very important. The hand postures are called *mudras* and there are many of them. As pure meditation places extreme emphasis on tension freedom, however, we only use two of the classic postures that require no tension in hands or arms as others do.

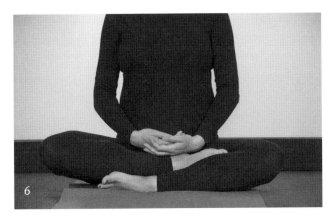

The first is one I call the butterfly *mudra* (see Photo 6). With palms facing up, one hand is cupped restfully on the other as if you are holding a delicate butterfly. Then the hands are just rested in your lap.

For the other position, the hands-cupped posture (see Photo 7), you simply rest the palms of your hands cupped on your knees.

You will find these *mudras* natural and comfortable, which is why Zen masters have used them for centuries.

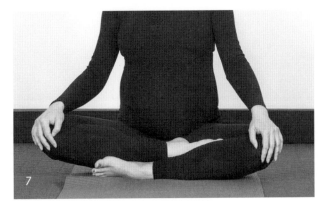

Meditating if you are unwell

As you probably know, there can be periods of time in your pregnant life in which you are not going to be feeling like climbing Mount Everest. Morning sickness with nasty nausea is a reasonably common experience for a little while.

Understandably, quite often the last thing an unwell mom-to-be wants to do is get onto the floor and meditate. In the event of your being unwell, however, keeping up meditative practice can be hugely beneficial (we'll talk more later about letting go tension and right breathing). Just remember that all exercises can be done while lying down—in bed if necessary.

The journey ahead

We are about to commence our journey by practicing some natural core skills that I call the Three Essences: letting go tension, 'right' or natural breathing, and quieting the mind. These practices teach us to become still of being and are necessary to help us create a lovely serene space within which we can dwell in tranquil silence and calm peacefulness. That dwelling is meditation.

I call the Three Essences the 'ancient arts' because they have been taught by yogis and Zen masters from much earlier times. They are skills that you actually already know because you practiced them naturally from birth and as a young child. But, sadly, these natural gifts tend to get smothered by the busyness and worries of trying to survive in contemporary society.

So, the key activity in your practice will be spending time on the Three Essences to rebuild these indispensable skills. The wonderful aspect of practicing the Essences is that we don't have to practice for years to begin attaining benefits. From the first moment of the very first exercise, the benefits have already begun.

CHAPTER FOUR

The First Essence: letting go tension

The profound level of freedom from tension needed for true wellbeing is based on the core principle of letting go—the basis of meditation at all levels. That starts, not by learning how to relax, but by practicing letting go tension until you can reach into, and sustain, the tension-freedom of a blissfully sleeping baby, just as you once could. Experiencing this level of tension-freedom is infinitely beyond any normal concept of relaxing.

In Zen meditation, we speak of three kinds of tension: natural, unnatural and stored tension. The first, natural tension, is the use of energy stored in our muscles ready to make the countless millions of body movements that enable us to function normally, from opening our eyes to running for the bus. When called upon, our muscles use the energy to create tension, which is converted to movement. Natural tension is good tension because, if we didn't have it, we would just fall over.

Unnatural tension (as in, not usual) is the same as natural tension except that it is held in the muscles for a longer period than required in normal use and then, after a period of time, is let go again. This happens as a result of the muscle action being driven by a stimulus such as anger, pain, jealousy, fear or even excitement.

The body systems gradually settle back to normal when the initial cause of unnatural tension is no longer present. Mostly, this kind of tension can also be regarded as a good tension because it is part of our body's natural, adrenalin-charged preparation for action or endurance (the fight-or-flight response).

Stored tension, within the meditative context, is seen as the long-term internalizing of (or holding on to) unnatural tension, rather than letting it go. The carrying of unnatural tension for a long period of time is so damaging that it eventually seems to become a normal part of you. It is tension most usually caused by negative emotions such as deep, ongoing anger, grief, guilt, fear, apprehension of the unknown, long-term lack of recognition or reward or, failure to meet expectations. I say, metaphorically, this kind of tension is 'stored in your bones' and carried as a destructive inner load.

Stored tension slowly becomes a permanent burden, damaging the very foundation of one's wellbeing. Stored tension is bad tension because it manifests as unhappiness and suffering. It can have a profoundly negative effect on our physical and psychological health, as well as on the very way we behave, conduct our lives and interact with others.

From a meditative point of view, I believe strongly that stored tension is the root cause of most illnesses and diseases, both physical and mental. This opinion is now being scientifically reinforced worldwide.

Accordingly, the first step on your meditation journey will be practicing letting go tension—the First Essence. Even if you decide not to go further than this first step, you will have given yourself a wisdom gift that will be of value, if you practice it regularly, for the rest of your life.

The practice of letting go tension

We have all spent a lifetime holding tension in our bodies to the point where we don't even realize we are doing it any more. There is little purpose then in saying 'just relax' to make your tension suddenly dissolve, because most people wouldn't know where to start. So, we commence our meditation journey with relearning this once-familiar skill in appropriate little baby-steps.

This first exercise is to help you experience just being quiet and still, which may be a fresh and luxurious new concept for you.

Note: Be aware that when practicing deep tension-freedom, you may find that the baby stops moving for a while. In meditation, this is not considered abnormal in any way, but if it continues and you are concerned, naturally contact your doctor.

EXERCISE 1

Resting calmly

› *Lie down comfortably in* savasana *(refer to Photo 1) with eyes closed.*
› *Allow your body to soften into the mat and just begin to . . . rest awhile.*
› *After a few minutes, you will become aware that your body is really still.*
› *This is a lovely point to start.*
› *Just endevor to melt into the feeling of resting calmly.*

Completing exercises and meditation

There is a right way to complete exercises and meditation so that you 'don't spill the calm' when you finish. (This is a lovely little phrase to repeat to yourself whenever you need to.) Ending an exercise in the right way enables the benefits of each practice to begin to be carried over into your daily life, one of the key aspirations of meditation.

The key to right completion is to always finish a practice very slowly and gently. Never jump up suddenly because you will be disoriented and instantly wipe out the invaluable calmness you are experiencing. A golden rule to take with you through all practices is, the longer the exercise or practice, the longer you take to complete it.

Right completion

> *Keep your eyes closed during completion so your awareness is in your body.*
> *Tell yourself that you are soon to finish your practice.*
> *When you are ready, take a deep, slow breath.*
> *Begin to move your fingers and toes, just a little.*
> *Next, move your hands and feet, followed by arms and legs, all very slowly.*
> *Then indulge in a slow, deep stretching of the body, just as a cat does.*
> *Having stretched, open your eyes and slowly sit up.*

Taking the calmness with you

After each practice, sit for awhile, reflecting on the experience you have just enjoyed. When you leave to go about your day, continue moving slowly and gracefully. This will help you to take the calmness with you until it becomes natural again.

The natural tension barrier

After you have practiced resting calmly for a week or so, you may think that you've 'got this relaxation stuff nailed'. You are definitely on your way, but the reality is that you can go much further—in fact, about 75 percent more.

We actually have a natural tension barrier beyond which, under normal circumstances of resting, your body will not let you relax any further. Your body has been trained over your lifetime to hold a certain level of tension so it is always primed for action. Even just sitting in a chair without falling off or being relaxed in front of the television requires body-tension. So, although you may feel relaxed in your first practices, you are in fact enjoying only about a quarter of your body's true capacity for deep tension-freedom.

The key to accessing true stillness is practicing a yogic technique of breaking through the body's natural tension barrier to reach the magical point of no tension at all. We do this by creating a false level of tension that is greater than the natural level. As this false level of tension is not familiar to the body, it will become confused as to just where the natural level is and will forget the natural tension point.

This is exactly what you want to achieve so that when you begin to practice letting go tension, you are able to just melt through the old barrier level into increasingly deeper levels of body stillness.

This next exercise is simple, but very important. Practice it until it becomes second nature. Being more tension-free than you have ever experienced before will be profoundly beneficial throughout your entire motherhood journey.

EXERCISE 2

Breaking through the natural tension barrier

› *Lie down in* savasana *as before, melting yourself into body restfulness.*
› *When you are as relaxed as you think you can be, slowly stiffen your entire body.*
› *Tense every muscle from head to toe at the same time. Screw up your face and make your hands into tight fists.*
› *When you have tensed the muscles throughout your body, hold this*

whole-body tightness for 10 to 15 seconds (you can count if you wish).

› *Then, almost imperceptibly, begin letting go the tension evenly throughout your whole body at the same time.*

› *Importantly, take about a minute for this very slow letting go.*

› *Focus on the feeling of tension seeping from you (one of the most beautiful experiences in the entire meditation journey).*

› *Continue releasing until you have let go as much tension as possible.*

› *Then just lie on your mat for five minutes or so, absorbed in the feeling.*

› *Begin to increase the 'lying absorbed' time a little each day until you are resting in this body-quietness for about 10 minutes.*

› *Complete as you have previously—slowly.*

Notes:

› *Never stiffen your body to the point of discomfort. If you are just beginning this exercise later in your pregnancy, the stiffening process can be very gentle—but still over the whole body. If you are well into your pregnancy, you can do this exercise equally well sitting up, either against a wall with cushions or in a lounge chair.*

› *If you feel you have let go too quickly, just start once more. If you don't let go very slowly, you will just relax back to the natural tension level.*

› *In each day of practice, hold the whole-body tension for a few seconds less than you did the previous day and take a few seconds less to let it go completely until you are holding the full tension only for some five seconds and then releasing it over about 30 seconds.*

› *Soon you will start at the natural tension level without tensing up at all.*

Directing your mind-focus

Now that you have broken through the tension barrier and relaxed as far as you think you can, you are still only about halfway towards being completely tension-free.

The next phase is to practice letting go even more tension by deliberately directing your mind-focus around your body to release even more tension literally from one end of your body to the other. This is quite an exhilarating mini-journey for all you tense ones!

The right place to start—an ancient secret

I will share an ancient yogic secret with you taught to me by my first master, Yogi Bashayandeh. Contrary to popular yoga teaching, in authentic Zen meditation you never start a tension-freeing practice by giving attention to your feet first.

Instead, we commence with the muscles around the eyes— always! The reason is simple. By letting go tension in the little muscles around your eyes, extraordinary things happen to your body. The very moment you start letting go tension in the muscles there, your whole body will begin letting go about another 20 or 30 percent of its tension. You can't help it, because it is an autonomic response. Then, quite amazingly, you will also find your breathing begins slowing down, again because you can't help it. The wonderment of slow breathing is that it adds a further deep layer of calmness over your whole body.

You only need to try it once to understand why we will start every practical exercise and later, meditation itself, with this yogic secret.

The next level of tension freedom

From now on, I will use the term 'bring your mind's focus (or awareness) to . . .', when asking you to give full attention to a specific part or area of your body. In doing so, you will become deeply conscious of nothing else but that area, as if your whole mind is just in that place.

If your mind wanders, just keep bringing your attention back to your area of focus and continue. This is one of the key principles for your entire journey: keep bringing any wandering attention back to 'just this'.

EXERCISE 3

The quieting

> *Settle into* savasana *and tense your whole body but only for two or three seconds before commencing the ever-so-gentle sinking through your tension barrier until you are as tension-free as you can be. Now the magic starts!*

> *Bring your 'mind's focus' to your closed eyes and then to the muscles around them. Attend to the little muscle groups such as under your eyebrows, then to the side of your eyes and under them. Deliberately let go tension in each little area one by one.*

> *Almost miraculously, you will feel a quite physical sense of the tension leaving those muscles. Keep your attention on one little area at a time.*

> *After you have given attention to your eyes, move your focus to your forehead, scalp and face and let go the tension there.*

> *Apply the same process of mind-focusing and letting go tension through the rest of your body but . . . working down your body, from head to toe, never the other way around.*

> *So, shift your focus from your face to neck, letting go all tension. Then move from the neck to the shoulders, down the arms, chest, tummy and then your back, until you have moved mind-awareness down the whole body to your toes, little by little, letting go tension as you travel.*

Melting chocolate

The final step in reaching profound tension-freedom is once more broadening your mind-focus to the whole body and doing a final, all-over 'let-go', much as you did at the beginning.

› *Imagine yourself melting into the mat and across the floor—as if you are chocolate melting out in the sun—as if letting go the 'boundaries' of your body.*

› *Rest your mind in this beautiful tension-free state for five minutes or so, or as long as you wish to enjoy it.*

› *Complete very slowly and enjoyably. Then as always—just sit for a bit.*

Notes:

› *Give considerable attention to mastering the skill of letting go tension. The effects can be powerful and positive for both you and your little one throughout pregnancy, but particularly in labor and delivery.*

› *When you feel ready, you can let go the initial tensing up (forever) and just begin letting go from the level of tension you are holding naturally when you lie down.*

› *Whenever you feel tense or agitated out there in the world, just stop and let go the tension around your eyes for a minute. Your whole body will relax—because you won't be able to help it. That is a wonderful gift you can take with you wherever you are.*

› *Increasingly, you will begin to discover that the calm you have experienced in the exercise will begin to last after you have walked away from your formal practice. As your days of practice pass into weeks and then into months, the sense of whole-being calmness derived from each session will begin to extend further and further across your day and into your general life activities.*

Letting go in the sitting position

This next important step is practicing everything you have been doing to date, but in a sitting posture (or any of the postures described earlier, depending on your preference and condition at the time).

In effect, the entire practice of the First Essence while sitting is identical to that which you have been practicing while lying down in *savasana*, except that now you will be holding a little tension in your back and balancing your head in a relaxed way.

As you are familiar with the phases of letting go body tension, I will not describe them in full again, but will just guide you more briefly to emphasize a few important points of practicing while sitting.

EXERCISE 4

Letting go tension while sitting

› *Take up the* sukhasana *posture (see page 32) or another of your choice. Close your eyes.*
› *After letting go tension in the whole body as before, then move to the muscles around your eyes first (as in the quieting phase). Take your mind-focus slowly down your body, exactly as you have been practicing.*
› *Give special attention to your back. Starting from the nape of the neck, very slowly let go tension, working all the way down to your buttocks. You will feel the tension gradually seeping from your back until it is relatively deeply tension–free, except that you are still sitting exactly as you were when you commenced—perfectly balanced.*
› *As before, move your awareness to just 'melting across the floor'.*
› *Complete slowly as you have been, including a stretch. Then just sit awhile.*

Notes:
› *In reality, you can let go about 80 percent of the muscle tension held in your back without your body moving a single millimetre.*
› *This is not very difficult at all. It is all about comfortable balance.*

That's how birds are able to sleep on one leg at night with their head under a wing. They have mastered the ability to hold perfect balance using just enough natural tension where needed.

Just sinking into tension-freedom

Until now, I have guided you through the different phases of letting go tension step by little step, like stepping stones across a creek. After you have become really familiar with each of the practice steps, from resting calmly to melting chocolate, however, it is time to begin to let go the steps themselves. (Remember, the whole art of mastering meditation is about letting go.)

In this next exercise, you simply allow each phase to just gently and fluidly flow into the next phase and then the next.

EXERCISE 5

Letting go the steps

› *So, in* sukhasana, *with your eyes closed, commence easing the tension from your body.*
› *At the same time, allow your mind-focus to drift to the muscles around your eyes, deeply letting go tension there.*
› *Fluidly run your mind in tension-freeing mode down your body without stopping at each little area. It becomes like a slow wave high on the beach whooshing gently back down to the water's edge.*
› *Then just drift your awareness into melting chocolate. Sit with it and complete when ready.*

Notes:

› *For a few practices, you will probably find that your mind continues to follow the different steps. Soon, though, the flow of one to the other will become just a single motion – a beautifully natural tension release without much effort at all.*

> The aim of this First Essence is to be profoundly, blissfully tension-free. With time and practice, you will develop the ability to just do it without thoughtful effort, which is wonderful for your wellbeing.

Letting go tension in a specific area

In the following exercise, the idea is to maintain your natural (ordinary) body tension while being sufficiently competent at becoming free of tension in just one specific area of your body.

I highly recommend that you give extra attention to this practice until you can do it at will, particularly for moments when you might be experiencing pain, such as at the time of giving birth. For that reason, it is an essential skill to develop.

Practice letting go tension selectively until it is almost second nature to you.

EXERCISE 6

Selective letting go

> In your sitting posture (or lying down if you wish) close your eyes and 'just rest' as you practiced in your first exercise—in other words, you retain the natural tension in your body.
> Now move your awareness to any one part of your body—say, your left hand. Bring deeply focused awareness to it. Begin to let go the tension there but nowhere else.
> Hold tension-freedom there for a minute or so before just slowly moving your fingers until your hand is back to normal tension.
> Then try this exercise in different areas of your body.
> But . . . begin to give particular and specific attention to your tummy and lower tummy areas. Include these areas in all practices and sometimes do this exercise just focusing on those areas.
> To complete, just begin to bring some normal tension back to the areas on which you've been practicing by moving a little before getting up.

EXERCISE 7

Letting go tension—with eyes open

After several days, try practicing exactly the same technique with your eyes open, wherever you are. For example, you may be just sitting in your kitchen having a cup of tea.

› *Just sit for a few moments and let go the tension in, say, your shoulders or your tummy.*
› *The effort then is to become aware when you are being distracted from the practice by, say, the flower in the vase or the cup in your hand. Keep bringing your focus back to 'just this'—letting go tension.*

Notes:

› *You may find this practice a little difficult initially because, with your eyes open, there are so many distractions around you. Just be patient. You will soon be able to focus just as well as with your eyes closed.*
› *This exercise is included so that in the flurry of, say, getting to the birthing place, or the busyness of people chatting and bustling about while you settle in there (and even later), you have another technique to help you come back to 'just this' and focus calmly on yourself.*
› *As you practice letting go tension over the coming weeks, you will begin to find that all the phases of the First Essence just seem to sweetly blend into a singular completeness of letting go. Not only that, you will find that it happens more quickly and naturally. You will just know where your body tends to hold its tension and be able to move in to offer relief.*
› *As you go on, the whole practice of the First Essence will seem to become a gentle continuum without deliberate effort. The several steps of letting go tension will have melded into one.*

Experiences and effects of letting go tension

From the beginning of practicing letting go tension, you may experience one of several physical reactions, feelings or experiences that, at first, may seem strange or even slightly discomforting. It is important to know that any unusual experience you may have while letting go tension is, in fact, natural and harmless because you are simply lying or sitting on a mat relaxing as purely as a newborn.

Therefore, any little experience at all is just a small sign that you are on the right track. It will soon pass as you deepen into stillness.

Some possible experiences include:

* Nerves or muscles jumping or twitching unexpectedly, like a fish suddenly leaping from a pond. Jumpiness or twitching indicates that the nerves and muscles are not receiving the familiar tension instructions from the brain. This is a good sign that you are letting go tension.

* Skin tingling or perhaps becoming warm. This is a very good reaction because it is the result of improved blood flow throughout the body and, particularly, to the skin.

* The sensation of floating or flying. If this happens and makes you feel uncomfortable, just open your eyes and reorient yourself. When you have settled, begin again or complete for the day.

* Feeling either really big or really small. In other words, as you begin to quieten your sensory awareness, you lose the normal sense of your body's proportion. You may feel as though you are blending into the environment. Know that you are not numb or paralysed, just slipping into a pleasurable state of deeper physical stillness. It is another sign that your practice is on track.

The benefits of tension-freedom

If you practice letting go tension daily, you will find that there are innumerable immediate and ongoing benefits. Even after just a few weeks of practicing, you may feel some improvement in your general wellbeing. In letting go negative tension, you release your body's natural calmness that wells up from within to flood the empty space once occupied by tension.

Emotional relief

Through your recent practicing of keeping your mind focused on your body, you have, in fact, begun the practice of mindfulness—the yogic art of having your mind present, right here, right now. When your mind is present, your thoughts are much less intrusive and the emotions attached to them are also reduced in intensity.

Gradually, as you become more practiced, emotions such as anxiety, apprehension or even fear will begin to melt away as body calmness takes over. This can be of immense temporary relief and a great resource to have in your expectant-mom kitbag!

Slowing metabolism

Just letting go tension throughout your body has the effect of slowing down your whole metabolism (much as a bear does while hibernating through the depths of winter). It lowers your blood pressure and slows your heart rate.

In deeper meditation, you can develop sufficient control over your body to achieve these body benefits virtually at will. This can be particularly useful for expectant moms who may have some blood pressure difficulties. Indeed, many people suffering from high blood pressure have been sent to the Meditation Sanctuary by their medical practitioners for this very reason. Through daily practice, most of them either substantially reduced or completely eliminated the need for medication.

More graceful movements

You may also begin to notice a greater natural fluidity and gracefulness in your movements simply because your body becomes less taut as you let go stored tension.

Renewed energy

On completing sessions of becoming tension free, you may experience feeling wonderfully renewed or energised. Holding your body tight with tension gobbles up energy and can be quite exhausting. Letting go tension therefore allows your natural energy to flow freely again. When you realize that your energy is a renewable resource simply attained by practicing the release of tension, you can begin to practice brief letting-go sessions for an energy boost whenever you need one.

Pain relief

When you reach complete body stillness, you may find that you are not feeling any of your usual aches or pains. That is not to say the causes of your muscle soreness, for example, are not still there but, just at the moment, you are not feeling them. As you progressively let go tension, you are slowing down the messages from the nerves and muscles throughout your body to the brain—and that includes the messages relating to pain. When you are meditatively tension free, those messages virtually cease.

Directed pain relief

Today meditation is used clinically worldwide for pain relief. As you increase your ability to direct your mind-focus, you are beginning to develop control over your body. You can already start using the techniques of letting go tension quite specifically for relieving various muscular and other pains.

This is an invaluable meditative skill for you to practice and hold onto for later on. Remember Vanessa who, between painful contractions, was actually able to fall asleep! She did it the following way, which you too can try whenever you feel pain of any kind.

Relieving pain

* Let go tension in your whole body as you know how (already this will provide some relief).

* Then direct your mind-focus to the unhappy area in your body.

* Focus deeply on it by placing your mind-awareness right in the middle of it (just as you can take your mind-awareness to, say, the muscles around your eyes).

* Then give attention to letting go tension in the painful spot or area until pain begins to subside. This is of particular value for headaches and migraines and can be of great value in pain-easing at birth.

It is a good idea to start practicing early in your pregnancy if possible so it is a mastered and worthwhile meditative practice against pain for you to use when necessary.

The 'afterglow'

Some of the deeper feelings you may experience as you nurture the art of letting go tension are a physical peacefulness and a sense of joy or blissfulness far superior to any effect achievable by any other form of relaxation. This 'afterglow' of wellbeing may only last a few minutes early on in your journey but, as you progress, the effect becomes increasingly long lasting and without conscious effort.

For this reason, it becomes increasingly important that you don't just consider your meditation experiences as nice while they lasted and then let them go the moment you walk out the door, allowing any benefits to be overtaken by the busyness of . . . next! This defeats the purpose of your practice. Gradually go beyond just sitting and practicing the exercises in your sanctuary by letting go tension wherever you are and whenever you think of it (even if it is just around your eyes or in your tummy).

It is now time to add the calming art of the Second Essence, right breathing, to your new skills, which is like having two scoops of calmness instead of one!

CHAPTER FIVE

The Second Essence: natural breathing for calmness and wellbeing

Breathing properly is particularly vital for expectant moms because you are looking after the wellbeing of two lives, not just one.

Breathing is the vital element of your existence because each breath imbues you with what the ancient yoga philosophers of India called *prana* (or the Chinese Zen masters, *chi*)—the 'life-force'. They taught that *prana* or *chi* is ever-present as energy manifested in your life and wellbeing. You absorb it when you breathe, eat, drink and expose your body to a sensible amount of sunshine. The skill is to relearn how to optimise this resource.

In many antenatal centres, various approaches to breathing are offered to the expectant mom, particularly during labor and then the birth itself. My intention in guiding you in meditative breathing and the practical way of using these techniques is not to say that you must or should replace other approaches. But I do recommend that you at least practice meditative breathing because it is natural and is proven to be of immense value throughout pregnancy and then, particularly, during labor and birth.

My strong advice, though, is to avoid vigorous breathing techniques such as strenuous panting. Such popularly taught breathing methods for birth actually diminish, rather than replenish, your energy as you go along.

This chapter will focus on the immense benefits of breathing naturally again, just as you could when you were born. Firstly, we'll look at how to renew your natural breathing to add another layer of calmness. Then we'll see how natural breathing can become an invaluable tool for you to draw on as a genuine (non-drug) antidote during times of anxiety, stress and apprehension throughout your motherhood journey.

Unhealthy breathing habits

At birth we knew how to breathe perfectly. Gradually, the anxieties and busyness of modern life have caused virtually the whole population to forget how to efficiently draw nourishment from the precious life-force that is available to them every moment of their existence.

As most people hold high levels of tension in their bodies most of the time, we resort to shallow breathing. In effect, we just use the top of our lungs to breathe and this eventually becomes normal. Just about everybody takes in about 16 shallow breaths a minute. The meditative person, however, when not meditating, just breathing naturally, will take in about four—and approximately twice the life-giving oxygen of the poor breather. That's twice the energy for half the effort!

From an emotional point of view, shallow rapid breathing is a reflection of an anxious, tense being. On the physical side, if you are just using your upper lungs, you are also not effectively eliminating toxins that build up in the lower lungs. At the same time, you are limiting the intake of *chi* (oxygen energy) that is available if you used more of your lungs with every breath, just as a baby does naturally by about six months of age.

Most people have simply forgotten how to breathe.

The benefits of natural breathing

Almost everyone, however, manages to potter along with shallow breathing. It is not as if we are falling like flies in the streets, so why bother making and maintaining an effort to change?

To begin with, the additional, deep calming effect induced by naturally rhythmic breathing dramatically reduces—and, indeed, can eliminate—the effects of stress such as anxiety. Almost immediately, you will also have more energy and a greater clarity of mind simply because the brain gets more oxygen—and so does your little one.

Consistent, deep natural breathing can also settle emotional swings and reduce negative emotions because energising your body more fully with oxygen automatically leads to you feeling far more positive, alert and alive. Breathing correctly also lessens nose, throat and lung congestion.

When you begin to breathe naturally as a matter of habit, your internal organs automatically receive better nourishment. The additional oxygen also purifies your bloodstream. You'll notice that the whites of your eyes become clearer and your skin will develop a healthier and more youthful appearance. Your lungs become more elastic and your chest and stomach muscles more supple. Right breathing also helps to reduce blood pressure and to top it all off, the taking in of all that life-force can strengthen your immune system and help to prevent or delay the onset of disease.

Perhaps most important of all for pregnant women, these benefits also flow to the baby in your belly.

Most people spend most of their lives essentially unaware of their breathing, let alone being transfixed by the wonderment of it. We shall begin then with a few little practices to reawaken your awareness to this simple fact.

EXERCISE 8

Becoming aware of your breathing

I have said that whenever you begin any meditative practice, you always prepare yourself by practicing the Essences first. In commencing this new practice, therefore, you start with letting go tension, the First Essence.

› *Sit in* sukhasana, *close your eyes and spend a few minutes letting go tension until you are calm.*
› *When you are tension free, take your mind-focus to your breathing.*
› *Spend a minute or two just becoming aware of your chest gently rising and falling.*
› *When your mind is focused on the rhythm of your breathing, start counting your in-breaths and out-breaths silently in your mind.*
› *So, after each breath in, count 'one' in your mind. Then after you breathe out, count 'two'.*
› *Continue to do this for two or three minutes.*
› *The next phase is to hold awareness on your breathing but stop counting.*
› *Maintain your focus on the action of breathing in and out without counting for several minutes.*
› *When you are ready, complete the whole practice session—slowly.*

EXERCISE 9

Deepening breathing awareness and focus

> *Again, practice through the First Essence, until tension free.*
> *Move your focus to being aware of your breathing but don't count.*
> *When you have settled into the rhythm of your breathing, take your mind-awareness to just inside the tip of your nose.*
> *Become aware of the cool air moving into your nostrils as you inhale and feel the warm air coming out as you exhale.*
> *Then move your awareness away from your nose and back to just focusing on the rise and fall of your chest.*

Returning to this basic awareness prepares you for the next phase, which is to become aware of your lungs themselves.

> *When you are ready, begin to imagine your in-breath as a color. (I like to visualize life-force as a rich, golden color.)*
> *So, when you breathe in now, visualize breathing in golden air (for example) and imagine it's swirling into your lungs. Then 'see' the golden air passing back through your nostrils as you breathe out.*
> *Do this about 10 to 20 times.*
> *To complete this exercise, gently let go imagining the color and take your awareness back to your chest gently rising and falling once more—then complete.*

Notes:

> *In authentic meditation, we breathe both in and out through our nose. The reason for nose breathing is simple. Your nasal passages are beautifully designed with tiny hairs called cilia that filter impurities from the air as you breathe in, reducing the amount of rubbish that cakes the linings of your lungs. So, nose designed for inhaling and exhaling, mouth designed for other things.*
> *If you over-breathe, either too deeply or rapidly, you may feel tingly, lightheaded, dizzy or see floaty spots before your eyes. None of*

these reactions is harmful, but if any occur, immediately slow your
breathing and start drawing more shallow breaths until you are back
to normal.

Mastering your breathing

This skill is invaluable for both labor and delivery. It is from this moment that the practice of right breathing begins and there is no longer any need to continue through all the little awareness exercises you've just practiced.

The first step in mastering your breathing is the practice of slowing it down. There are two reasons for this. Firstly, as your metabolism begins to slow down as a result of letting go tension, less and less energy is required—so less breathing is required. Secondly, the slower the breathing, the calmer you become.

Because your body's need for oxygen varies according to energy demand, you can actually learn to modulate the pace of your breathing according to your body's requirement. For meditating, you can learn to reduce the pace of your breathing substantially, like animals hibernating. If your body needs extra energy under exertion, such as during delivery, you can practice a technique to maximize your oxygen intake without resorting to rapid, shallow, energy-sapping panting.

EXERCISE 10

Slowing the rhythm

› *Settle into your posture and practice tension-freedom for a few minutes.*
› *Take your mind-awareness to your breathing. Hold until your focus is settled there.*
› *Begin to count the seconds it takes to breathe in and out.*
› *Begin to consciously control your breathing by increasing the time*

taken for each breath. Deliberately set a count of about two (seconds) more than you were taking before. For example, if you were taking three to breathe in and three out, try taking five in and the same out.

› *Continue counting to the slower pace until it is comfortable.*

› *When you are ready, you can stop counting—just focus on the slow rise and fall of your chest for several minutes before completing.*

Notes:

› *When you slow your breathing, don't take in any more air than you were. Just breath in the same amount as before, but more slowly. You will find that adding just a couple of extra seconds to your normal breathing rate is quite comfortable in the early stages.*

› *Just slowing your breathing to, say, five seconds both in and out means that you are breathing about six times a minute, already a long way from shallow breathing at 16 or so cycles a minute.*

› *Every week or two, endeavor to add about one more second to both the in and the out breath until you reach about eight to 10 seconds in and out. You will then have slowed your breathing cycle, quite naturally, to about three or four per minute—perfect for creating deeper calmness.*

› *Whenever you think of it, practice slowing your breathing as you go about your daily activities.*

Right or natural breathing

Imagine that your lungs are divided into three segments (lower, middle and top). Most people only use about a third of their lung capacity. In other words, they only breathe into the top third of their lungs. Leaving the remaining segments of the lungs out of action means that they become rubbish dumps for accumulated toxins which, in turn, have a seriously negative effect on your wellbeing.

Instead of experiencing oxygen-enriched vitality, which you really need during your pregnancy, the body spends much of its precious energy resources trying to eliminate toxicity, hence the modern maladies of general tiredness, easy exhaustion, lack of motivation and significantly increased susceptibility to sickness and disease—none of which you need at this time.

Through right or natural breathing you simply relearn how to use your entire lung capacity the whole time, as a matter of habit, just as you did when you were a baby. We will practice relearning how to breathe right in three little steps. Firstly, tummy breathing (breathing into your lower lungs), which is the most vital. Secondly, breathing into your middle lungs, which will become increasingly important as your little one grows. Finally, the third step (upper lungs) is the way you have breathed for most of your adult life.

Hara breathing, or tummy breathing

Most westerners are totally unfamiliar with tummy breathing, but in Zen meditation it has been a core principle since ancient times. The ancient Chinese masters called the specific area just below your belly button *tan t'ien* (the field of heaven), because they believed this was the spiritual centre of their being.

Japanese masters call the general area of the mid/lower abdomen that rises and falls with correct tummy breathing the *hara*. They regarded it as a source of energy and they were right, of course. What they had really identified was the fact that breathing properly and using the whole lung capacity can provide you with a renewable source of energy. It provides you with healthy life itself. This enriching way of breathing needs to be practiced until it again becomes utterly natural.

EXERCISE 11

Practicing tummy, or hara, *breathing*

If you are already more than four months pregnant, leave this practice and move on to the next exercise.

Step 1

Take a small book with you to your meditation place. It will be used as a 'prop' shortly.

> *Lie down in the* savasana *position.*
> *Put one hand horizontally across your tummy, centred on your belly button and place the other by your side.*
> *Now deliberately take in a larger, longer breath, trying to take some air down into the lower lungs. This may force your tummy to rise.*
> *Continue gently practicing until your hand is moving up and down with each breath, even if only a little.*

When this happens, you are tummy (or *hara*) breathing, drawing air into your lower lungs that in turn expands them, forcing your tummy outwards a little. Gradually, of course, your pregnant tummy will expand, so you will modify this practice as you go further.

Step 2

> *After two or three minutes practicing with your hand on your tummy, place the book there instead and rest both hands, face down, beside you.*
> *In this naturally relaxed pose, try and push the book up and down a little with your* hara *breathing.*
> *When you notice your 'field of heaven' moving, take your mind-focus to that area. Become aware of the feeling of the air going in and out of your lower lungs and your tummy rising and falling. You can do it— but don't over-exert yourself or you may get a little dizzy.*

Step 3

> *After this practice becomes comfortable, the next step is to put the book aside.*
> *With your hands still face down beside you, just focus on the slow rising and falling of your tummy. Breathe slowly and gently for a few minutes.*
> *Practice* hara *breathing until you find it is feeling more natural.*

Note:

> *If the book keeps sliding off your tummy because it is already of a 'certain shape' (the tummy, not the book), leave the book aside without trying to force your tummy out any further. You will actually find the middle chest area expanding a little sideways quite naturally as you begin to breathe around your growing baby.*

EXERCISE 12

Hara *breathing in your meditation (sitting) posture*

The next step in returning to natural breathing is practicing exactly what you have just been doing while lying down, but now in the sitting posture.

> *Sitting quietly, let go tension first, as always, before moving your awareness to your breathing.*
> *Slow your breathing and just immerse yourself in the calmness.*
> *Place your hand horizontally across your tummy with the centre of your hand resting over your belly button.*
> *Try taking air into your lower lungs as you did before, pushing your tummy out just a little.*
> *Breathe out slowly, allowing your hand to move back in as your tummy deflates.*
> *When you are able to do this comfortably, take your hand away from your tummy and rest both of them in your mudra.*
> *Focus your mind on the gentle in and out movement of your 'field of heaven'.*
> *Enjoy the higher level of calmness you will experience before completing slowly when ready.*

EXERCISE 13

Rhythm or full-lung breathing

There is a beautiful, calming, natural rhythm to the way you once breathed. Rhythm breathing means consciously and efficiently using your entire lungs to breathe, not just the top part of them. Although this is an optimal, natural way of breathing, it is not critical for meditation—it just adds another layer of calmness.

You have been practicing expanding your lower lungs with your in-breath while it is still comfortable to do so. The next step is to consciously expand the middle segment of your lungs. In your early practice, this will be a noticeably separate step to your *hara* breathing until it becomes natural again.

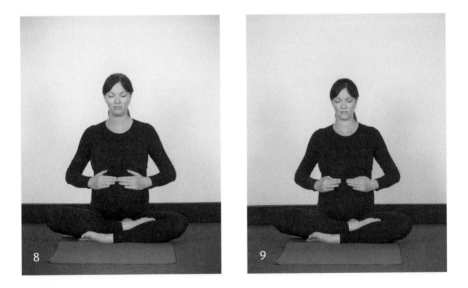

Mid-lung breathing
> *Place both hands horizontally on your lower rib cage (about one hand-width above where you had your hand for the start of tummy breathing) so the tips of the middle fingers are touching (as shown in Photo 8).*

> *The sequence now is to push your tummy out (taking air into the lower lungs) as before. Then draw in a little more air. This will go into the middle-lung area and expand it too. The endevor is to allow your ribs to expand out sideways.*

> *When you do this effectively, you will notice that the tips of your fingers are forced to part a little as the air in the middle section of your lungs expands your chest sideways (see Photo 9).*

> *As you breathe out, the tips of your fingers will come together.*

> *Then practice this exercise with your hands back in your mudra.*

As your tummy grows, your lower lungs will become more compressed and it will be increasingly difficult to *hara* breathe. Although you will naturally mid-lung breathe, it is good to become aware of and practice this skill so you don't resort to panting or shallow breathing, particularly later on when you will need optimal breathing practices.

Upper-lung breathing

The final step of the in-breath sequence is to become aware of using the top third of your lungs in the right way.

> *Fill the lower lungs (still pushing out your tummy), then the mid-section (ribs sideways), then breathe in a little more, expanding the top part of your lungs.*

> *The skill involved this time is not to raise your shoulders to take in more air. Instead, try and push your chest outwards (even if only a little) towards the wall opposite.*

> *Breathe out, letting all three segments of your lungs just naturally subside, making sure to empty the lower lungs (tummy pushed in a little).*

You may find it helpful to say 'lower . . . middle . . . top' in your mind as you breathe into each of the three areas one-by-one, gently filling them with *chi* and then smoothly breathing out the residue.

> Then with your hands in the mudra *again, practice this exercise in its full sequence.*
> *Let go your saying of 'lower . . . middle . . . top' and just focus on the whole rhythmic process, running the three actions of inhaling together as one smooth, fluid action.*
> *Whenever you are ready, try and slow your breathing a little more.*

Important:
> *Remember that your rhythm in-breath is a gentle, natural action and that you do not need to fill your lungs to the brim. In fact, when meditating, the whole sequence can be almost imperceptible because you are so calm and still.*

Breathing out properly

Up until now, you have been breathing out by collapsing the lungs, ensuring that the lower part feels empty. We shall now add the right breathing-out skill to ensure you completely rid yourself of stale, toxic air with every out-breath. It is really very simple. Babies can do it from about six months when their lungs are more developed. The natural way to breathe out is simply reversing the sequence of your in-breath.

> *After you take a full, in-breath (tummy out, ribs wide, top chest out), breathe out.*
> *Start by expelling the air from the lower part of your lungs first by pushing your tummy in as far as you can.*
> *Then, in order, close your ribs inwards as air leaves your middle lungs and then collapse the air from the top part of your lungs to complete the movement. Now your lungs have been completely emptied of stale air.*
> *Start the cycle over again, always filling the lower lungs first.*

Notes:
> *Do not worry if this exercise is difficult at first. Don't force it. Be patient and gentle with yourself, allowing the practice to become*

natural again. As I mentioned previously, later in your pregnancy that will mean being aware of, and using, mid-lung breathing rather than either hara or just shallow breathing.

› *To make it easier, follow your mind-instructions of 'lower . . . middle . . . top' until your body can remember the sequence. Then let go the mental chat so the words are not a distraction.*

› *Once you have practiced this rhythm for a while, your entire breathing movement will begin to feel like standing in the sea about chest deep and being gently moved by the rhythmic and soothing movement of the waves—deeply, beautifully calming and the perfect antidote to feeling anxious or apprehensive.*

EXERCISE 14

Practicing the first two Essences together

Before we lift the practice to another level, there is one more exercise to begin to master: practicing the first two Essences together from the very beginning of your sessions. This means starting to flow the letting go of tension quite naturally into the breathing practice without a pause between the first two Essences.

In effect, they become integrated, creating a natural base for soon practicing the Third Essence, stilling the mind, as well as becoming your natural prelude to all further exercises and meditation.

› *Before you begin letting go body tension, take in a slow, deep breath, starting with the lower lungs. Release it gently while, at the same time, you begin letting go the tension around your eyes.*

› *As you continue the slow breathing cycle, continue to let go tension throughout your body. (You will find that tension is more readily let go when breathing out.)*

› *Continue doing both until you have fully let go tension and reached your optimal pace of slow and deep breathing.*

› *Sink into this quietness of body and breathing, dwelling in the experience before completing.*

Notes:

> The effect of doing both Essences deliberately at the same time can be remarkable as they have a compounding effect. Practicing slow, deep breathing helps the tension-freeing process that, in turn, automatically assists the slowing of your breathing.

> The final aim of this practice is to be able to do it naturally without conscious effort. With practice, eventually the Three Essences (including stilling the mind) can be attained virtually simultaneously, with complete body, breathing and mind quietness being reached in just a few seconds. This is a most valuable and lovely natural skill to develop through your pregnancy and take with you into the birthing place.

Breathing practices for extra energy and endurance

Once you have practiced the key exercises of slowing and deepening your breathing, there are several further classic practices that you can take on board to enhance a sense of calmness and wellbeing. They enable greater control over your breathing while strengthening your lungs and abdominal muscles. All of them are of great value as your pregnancy matures, and particularly helpful for labor and birth.

EXERCISE 15

Whole-body breathing

Earlier, when we began breathing-awareness exercises, you practiced a lung-awareness exercise in which you imagined that the *chi* or life-force was a lovely color. I asked you to visualize it swirling around your lungs as you breathed in. This next exercise is similar, but now we take it a little further.

> Upon settling into your *hara* or *rhythm* breathing, begin to visualize the air being breathed in as a color.

› *This time, on your in-breath, try and visualize the colored air going beyond your lungs as though it is spilling over from them and flowing gently into your whole body. It is as if you are not just breathing into your lungs but into all of you.*

› *On your out-breath, visualize the colored air being drawn from your whole body, out via your nose and into the universe.*

› *Now, while drawing air into your whole body, let go visualizing the color. The visualization now becomes one of deeply focusing on taking in the life-force with each in-breath to nourish every cell in your body. The out-breath then takes the spent residue back out into the universe.*

› *You can add this practice to the first two Essences for about five minutes before completing.*

Notes:

› *There are helpful (and therapeutic) variations on this refreshing exercise. For example, you can visualize the air being taken in as wellbeing, nourishing your whole body.*

› *You can also visualize the* chi *as a sense of joy that you happily inhale with your in-breath. In due course, while actually engaged in this visualization, you may experience a remarkably freeing sense of wholeness, joy, peacefulness or wellbeing.*

› *Many students have mentioned to me that this very practice alone, and the sense of 'being at one' with your breathing it brings, seems to help in alleviating some of the heaviness of health and emotional difficulties. It is a deeply calming practice.*

EXERCISE 16

Dynamic breathing

Dynamic breathing is consciously breathing in and out using your entire lungs—lower, middle and top—all at the same time. It is a method of getting extra oxygen more quickly for times of exertion and when real endurance is called for, such as running a marathon or delivering a baby. (At that time, you most likely will only use your middle and upper lungs.)

Important:

Dynamic breathing is of particular importance to you because it will give you as much energy as rapid panting, but you only use about one-third of the energy-sapping effort required for panting. It is also a way of breathing that can enable you to remain much calmer under duress. This is a wonderful exercise to master because you can gently practice it anywhere, any time.

> *In your sitting posture, let go tension and focus on your breathing.*
> *Gradually take it to a slower pace.*
> *Through the nose, breathe in quite gently but try to breathe into all of your lungs at the same time.*
> *Exhale slowly through the nose but from all parts of your lungs at the same time.*
> *When this becomes comfortable, you can practice quickening the pace little by little.*
> *Finally, as the pace becomes more rapid, you can practice the whole exercise using open-mouth breathing out, or even using your mouth for both in- and out-breath if you feel the need.*
> *When this exercise is working comfortably, begin to practice all over again but, this time, while lying down in savasana, as you might when delivering your baby.*
> *After a few minutes, slow your breathing again to hara or mid-lung mode.*

Notes:

> *When the time comes, practicing dynamic breathing during contractions for example, and then slowing it back to hara or mid-lung breathing between contractions can be an effective way of dealing with pain and then quickly returning to restful calmness.*
> *While lying down for your practice, a helpful variation is to do*

the same but with your knees bent and your feet drawn up to your buttocks. A further variation is to practice gently while on your hands and knees (both potential birth positions).

› *Never practice any variation that is physically uncomfortable at any stage of your pregnancy.*

› *Do not over-breathe. If there is any discomfort such as lightheadedness, slow your breathing. Your body knows exactly how much energy it needs to cope with any situation so listen to it carefully, understand its messages and respond accordingly. This is much better than taking instruction and advice from others who are not in your body!*

EXERCISE 17

Breathing walks

A breathing walk is a short walk when your whole mind-focus is on your breathing and the action of walking itself, at the same time. It can be wonderful for breathing, strengthening and endurance, particularly if you are walking for two.

These walks in fact can develop into *kyo gyo*—walking meditation. This is not the usual little meander along when your mind thinks about anything and everything. It is being deeply aware of breathing and walking, breathing and walking. It is the meditative practice of physical mindfulness—giving attention to being just here, just now. It can be exhilarating and calming. Try to walk about three times a week, increasing the distance a little each time.

You can practice little spells of dynamic breathing while walking. Perhaps occasionally, you might walk for a while longer, which requires some extra exertion. When you begin to puff a little, begin consciously expanding and contracting your whole lungs at once. Breathing in this way will gradually ease the need to puff as you will be taking in plenty of *chi*, even for vigorous activity. Again, this is great preparation for later on.

Strengthening exercises

The following exercises are designed to gradually increase lung capacity, better eliminate toxins and further develop strength in the lungs and abdominal muscles. Please start them slowly, increasing the repetitions gradually. Do not extend yourself physically beyond your comfort level at any time.

I suggest you keep a record of your daily practice, starting each exercise with just one repetition on the first day and only moving to two after three days, three repetitions after another three days and so on (using your diary to help you here).

The aim is to build your strength slowly until you are doing these exercises for about seven minutes a day. You can practice them throughout your pregnancy, but do progress gently. When they become even slightly difficult, it is time to stop.

EXERCISE 18

Deep breathing—opening your lungs

If you are unable to stand for long, you can practice most of these exercises sitting on a chair or in bed.

STEP 1
› *Stand straight with your legs together and hands by your side.*
› *Gently let go any tension and introduce gentle hara breathing for a minute or so.*
› *Breathe in to a count of five while slowly lifting your arms straight out sideways away from your body until they are horizontal to your shoulders.*
› *Hold your breath for three seconds with your arms extended. Then slowly return them to your side, again counting to five while breathing out through your nose.*
› *When you are comfortable with the exercise, you can increase*

the counting, say to about seven or so, to slow the activity further.

STEP 2

› *The same as above, but keep raising your arms so they are held vertically over your head with your fingers touching and pointing towards the sky.*

› *Again, start with a count of five in and out. Pause at the top while holding your breath.*

› *Increase repetitions and time count as above.*

EXERCISE 19

Cleansing your lungs

STEP 1

› *While standing, put your hands on your hips and take a deep breath, filling your whole lungs, starting with your lower lungs. Do this on a slow count of five in.*

› *Then expel all the air as suddenly and as forcefully as you comfortably can through pursed lips (like a fish's mouth).*

› *Empty your lungs as completely as you can. Push your tummy in (gently) at the end to get rid of all the used air.*

› *Again, start with one only on the first day and increase slowly.*

STEP 2

› *Breathe in as for the last exercise but this time expel all the air in three separate, forceful puffs instead of one big out-breath. Make a tighter fish-mouth so your lungs have to work harder to force out the air.*

› *Make the last of the three puffs a longer, complete emptying breath. Again, push your tummy in gently.*

› *Repeat as before.*

EXERCISE 20

Strengthening your lungs and focusing

In yoga, this exercise is called 'bellow breathing'. You will automatically feel your chest and abdomen muscles getting a gentle workout.

STEP 1

› *Breathe in deeply through your nose. Hold your breath for a few moments and then force it out as slowly as possible through a very tight fish-mouth. (Your cheeks will puff out while you do this one.) This is great for the tummy muscles. Remember, gently as you grow.*

This next exercise is the yogic equivalent to panting but note that it is using *hara* breathing. Practice it more gently as you become bigger.

STEP 2

› *Breathe in and out quite forcefully and quickly through your nose by pushing the abdomen area in and out—slowly at first or you will pass out!*
› *Ever so gradually, develop the pace to about 30 per minute. (Yes, one 'in and out' every two seconds or so.) Always make your last exhalation a long, slow, relaxing one.*

Practice this exercise for only about five seconds the first day, building up to about 30 seconds over a few weeks, only for as long as it remains comfortable.

EXERCISE 21

Fun breathing practice . . . with a purpose

This is a fun way to strengthen your lungs, chest and tummy muscles. You need a candle and a lighter. It is also wonderful for children with asthma, but you must supervise them!

> › On the first day, place the lit candle close to your mouth and blow it out with one forceful breath using your fish-mouth. Just do it once on the first day.
> › Each day, move the candle a little further away before blowing it out. Slowly increase the number of times you do so.
> › Later, even though it will become too far to actually blow out, continue moving it further away to see if you can just stir the flame with your breath.
> › Feel the effort required from your chest and tummy muscles to blow it out.
> › Eventually you will be able to flicker the flame all the way across a room.

Active meditation

Active meditation means taking your developing skills with you as you go about your daily life. In Zen, we say that each moment is an opportunity to practice our skills such as letting go tension and/or slowing and deepening our breathing. To get the optimum benefit from your practice, try and develop a daily habit of little practices whenever you think of it.

The second aspect of active meditation is to make it genuinely active. Using the first two Essences in an integrated way can be a powerful meditative weapon. I call it the Samurai solution. It can be triggered into play on an as-or-when-needed basis such as during moments of stress or anxiety.

You can now unpack the letting go weapons and apply them to really helping you when emotions begin to fray or become overwhelming. At such times, the first really important step is to become truly aware of the negative feeling, even naming it.

The moment you begin to feel stressed though, is the precise moment to call on your meditative practices and apply them to induce calmness. At the moment of need, immediately close your eyes and take your mind-focus to the muscles around them and begin letting go tension as you have practiced. At the same time, begin to slow and deepen your breathing.

Just slipping quickly into tension-free mode around the eyes and slowing your breathing can offer quite rapid relief from stress and feelings of anxiety. This is not always easy to do but, with practice, it can become a natural and wonderful way of bringing you back to calmness.

CHAPTER SIX

The Third Essence:
calming the unquiet mind

It is our mind alone that causes our joys and our woes.

– ANCIENT YOGIC WISDOM

At the Meditation Sanctuary where I teach, students are asked to do some very simple exercises that reveal to them the way they actually think. They are asked to become aware of, and write down, every thought they have over a 15-minute period. They then underline thoughts relating to their past and their musings about the future.

They are asked to circle thoughts that are about the actual present such as 'I am hungry' or 'I like the music being played'. Then they are asked to place a plus symbol over all their positive thoughts and a minus symbol over all negative ones. Finally, they are asked to read over their writing again, thought by thought, and place a plus symbol over all their positive thoughts and a minus symbol over all negative ones.

Invariably, students are astonished by the secrets their writings reveal. They discover that they spend most of their time thinking about the past or the future, with relatively little time dwelling in the present. Further, they discover that they move from the past to the future or present and back again repeatedly, within a matter of seconds.

To their amazement, they also see how their emotions career rapidly and virtually out of control—from positive to negative as their thoughts shift—just while they are sitting without any stimulus from outside. Right before them, they have a snapshot of the way their mind works from the moment they wake up until they go to bed.

In summary, the vast majority of people—especially those who do not meditate—spend each day with their minds full of incessant, distracted, undisciplined, worry-based mental chatter. This is the main cause of stress and tension that, in turn, can lead to anxiety, fear and apprehension—the very last emotions you need to experience as an expectant mother. Of course, it is far preferable to be exactly the opposite: calm, clearly focused and able to master difficult situations. This is not as hard as it may seem, even after a lifetime of relatively mindless mental chattering.

So calming the unquiet mind, which then can give you an exceptional capacity to focus, is the most important of the three essential skills or Essences that, layered onto a tension-free body and combined with gentle breathing, can create an ideal state of mental restfulness.

The two steps to a still mind

Step i

The first step to a quiet mind is reducing the incessant babble to just one thought—a single point of focus.

There are many ways of achieving this single-pointed focus of the mind. I have chosen several of the more pure meditative techniques that are appropriately gentle, effective, soothing and beautiful.

I would like you to practice each one of them but, as you progress, you will find that one or two of the techniques are much easier for you than others. That is the time to let go the others and just practice your favourite ones until they become as natural to you as your morning cup of tea. Whatever technique you choose is as valid as any other—the purpose of all of them being to quieten those babbling thoughts to just a single point of focus.

When you develop this focusing skill, you will find it deeply calming, particularly as you prepare for delivery and during the birth. The greater your ability to focus your mind on just one fully dedicated point of focus, the greater value it will be because you essentially fill up all that mind-space previously devoted to apprehension and anxiety, with calmness.

STEP 2

The next step takes quietening the mind to another level—pure, restful stillness. Even though your mind is so much calmer when you have reached single-pointed focus than when the usual babble is filling it, it is not yet perfectly quiet. It is still full of the subject of the single-pointedness. So at the end of each technique, I will show you how to let it go so you can dwell in the calmness of a mind-silent serenity. Then you are really meditating.

By reaching into this meditative stillness each day, the calmness and awareness will gradually go beyond just sitting. It begins to spill across the rest of your waking day for increasingly longer periods. The eventual aim of the serious meditator is to sink into this state of mindful awakeness the whole time—because you can't help it. This return to an original naturalness is beautifully summed up in a student comment:

A friend said to me yesterday, 'You don't talk about doing meditation anymore. Why?' My response was, 'I don't talk about breathing either, do I?'

A word on 'experiences'

When you start meditating and your mind begins to free itself from the usual distractions, some little experiences may pop in to take up the emptying thought space. This may happen until your mind becomes familiar with the highly novel idea of just being still. Any unusual experiences in your practice are perfectly fine, harmless and normal. They are, in fact, little signposts that you are indeed practicing well – otherwise they wouldn't happen. They are all just little inner-body mental events resulting from the mind becoming quiet. As your practice deepens though, experiences begin to fade and then not appear at all.

Possible little experiences

- Your first awareness of a 'happening' is that your thoughts may seem to separate from you and just seem to be floating about 'out there' rather than 'in here'. As one student described it, 'I was aware of my thoughts, but they seemed to be in another room'.

- You may occasionally witness nebulous color-shapes or feel surrounded by colored light.

- Some experiences may be more vivid. Some people have 'visions', such as morphing faces, beautiful lights and iconic figures.

- You may hear sounds such as voices, music or chanting.

- You may also lose immediate perception of your body and feel quite disembodied as if you are not there. You may feel as if you are rising from the ground or floating in space.

Single-pointed focus using a mind mantra

The use of a mantra to quieten the mind to single-point focus is an ancient and classical technique practiced across many cultures. Its practice ranges from the repetition of a single word to the chanting of elaborate verses that usually have a religious connotation.

In the classical way, a mantra is most often spoken, chanted or hummed aloud. In authentic meditation, any word or phrase can be used as a mantra because it is not the word or phrase itself that is important, but the repetition of it.

For this exercise, I would like you to select a mantra, a personal word or phrase that you find soothing or lulling in your repeating of it. This will be the mantra you can use for awhile now, although you can change it whenever you wish. If you have difficulty in choosing one, try one of the following lulling word or phrases. The meaning of the words is immaterial to the effectiveness of your meditation.

Examples of word mantras

Ananda	Niyama
Nirvana	AUM
Samsara	OM
Samhara	

Examples of phrase mantras

I love rainbows

Lightness of being

Just this

Just now

I am silent and serene

I love you

EXERCISE 22

Practicing a mind mantra

› *Spend about 10 minutes reaching your essential stillness (tension-free body,* hara *breathing). This will build your base of calmness.*

› *Then introduce your chosen mantra.*

> Begin repeating it over and over so that you can hear it in your mind.
> Endevor to hold pure focus on the mantra for about two minutes, building that time a little each day.
> When you want to finish the practice, let go the mantra by taking your mind-focus back to your breathing and dwell on it for a minute or so.
> Slowly complete.

Notes:
> Sometimes while repeating your mantra you will find your attention lapsing, particularly at the beginning. This is normal in early practice, so just be patient.
> As soon as you become aware of thoughts popping in again, just take your attention back to listening to the sound of your mantra.
> The secret is to just keep bringing yourself back until gradually you'll realize that you're wandering away less and less.
> After a while, the repetitive sound of your mantra will seem to be just meaningless white noise. That is the idea and is, in itself, a calming, lulling place to be.
> Only move to the next exercise when you are able to focus quite fully on your mantra for several minutes.

EXERCISE 23

Letting go the mind mantra technique—beginning meditation

The aspiration now becomes letting go the distraction of a mantra ticking over in your mind, thus gentling it to an aware, perfect stillness.

> As before, progress through the Three Essences, bringing your mind to single-pointed focus with your mantra. Always take your time to do this.
> Give particular attention to it, until you are aware that your thoughts have largely disappeared into the lulling of your mantra.

> *Imagine your mantra is being played to you on a distant radio.*
> *Now turn the sound down in your mind, just as if you might turn down the sound using the volume knob on a radio.*
> *Importantly, do the turning down ever so slowly, almost imperceptibly, but keep listening to the sound of your voice saying the mantra even as it becomes progressively quieter and recedes into the distance.*
> *Keep listening until you are straining to hear the sound of the mantra as it gradually fades away entirely. You will be focusing on . . . silence.*
> *Soon enough, you will begin to experience an exquisite sense of calmness and stillness.*
> *Endevor to just sit, dwelling in the stillness.*
> *When you feel ready to complete, return awareness to your breathing and do so in the usual, graceful manner.*

The first time you experience not thinking, an amazing thing happens—you begin to think . . . as in 'Wow, I've done it!' That's perfectly fine. Bashayandeh told me that his first mind-opening dabble into true silence made him so excited he couldn't get back to meditation for a week. So, what to do?

> *When thoughts start, you simply turn up the mantra again and listen until you are once more absorbed in the sound of it.*
> *Repeat the turning down to silence all over again.*
> *Every time a thought comes in from then on, use the same process.*
> *Sit calmly for a while after completing.*

Notes:

> *Gradually, you will find that the time of quietness between thoughts begins to be noticeable, perhaps only a second or two at first. But then the thought-pause will progressively lengthen until the magic day when you are able to hold your attention on the silence, without thought at all, for minutes at a time—and then longer.*
> *When dwelling in pure silence, even for just a little while, you are then genuinely, tranquilly meditating.*
> *Soon you will begin to experience the initial after-effect of meditating—*

being very calm for a period following the practice. The more accomplished you become, the longer this calmness lasts, which is the actual purpose of doing all this. Be patient though—it takes time.

Moving to a new technique

You should only move to the practice of a new technique after you have reasonably accomplished the previous technique and are comfortable with it. You must also feel free to move to the next technique if the last one is defying your best efforts. That is not uncommon, it simply reflects the fact that we are all different and people find some techniques easier than others.

Be like water finding its way down a mountain. Follow the path (technique) of least resistance, the one that helps you most to find calmness of mind.

EXERCISE 24

The vocalised mantra

This is a classic, beautiful and effective practice that takes the using of a mantra a little further and one that I have enjoyed for many years.

Thousands of years ago, the Rishees (original yogis) understood that the whole universe is comprised of energy that vibrates. They believed that this vibration made a sound, which they are said to have experienced deep in their meditation. It is this sound that these men tried to reproduce as the word *AUM* (say aahh—ooo—mmm) which, in many practices, has become the very familiar *OM*.

When spoken softly out loud and chanted as a mantra, *AUM* (or *OM*) has two points of focus. Firstly, you listen single-pointedly to the soft sound and then you gradually shift your focus to the gentle, soothing vibration you feel in your body and head.

In this exercise, as you breathe out, your voice vocalises the mantra. The sound lasts for the duration of each, long out-breath. We'll start just using a hum and then move to a full *AUM* mantra that also reinforces your *hara* breathing at the same time.

› *Sink into your essential stillness.*
› *With mouth closed, begin to hum aloud for the duration of your out-breath. (Hum loudly enough so that you can hear yourself.)*
› *When you are ready, open your mouth on your out-breath and start saying AUM in the three parts as follows:*
  – *While breathing out, the first part of the AUM mantra is 'a' (pronounced 'aahh'). You say this slowly as you begin breathing out from your tummy (hara breathing).*
  – *Then the 'u' sound (pronounced 'oo' as in 'wool'). Your mouth is rounded like a fish and the sound seems to emanate from the middle of your lungs because, as you continue to breathe out, you are closing your mouth slowly in preparation for making the 'm' sound.*
  – *Then, when the sound of the 'm' follows, it is held with your mouth closed so the vibration ('mmm') resonates in the head and then throughout your whole body.*
› *Focus deeply on the vibration while saying 'mmm'.*
› *Repeat until you feel a deep calmness settling in your whole body and mind.*
› *To complete, just rest the sound, focusing on the gentle rhythm of your breathing.*

Notes:

› *AUM is a perfect word for extended, slow mantra expression because the three letters can be drawn out for as long as your out-breath lasts.*
› *After a while, a vocalised mantra feels as though you are massaging every cell in your body. It seems to permeate your whole being and brings with it an inner sense of great harmony and peacefulness that has natural health benefits. The practice is another valuable one for alleviating the symptoms of anxiety and depression.*
› *The lulling beauty of the sound and the sweet calming of the vibration are also felt and heard by your baby and become another way in which she becomes increasingly familiar with you while still in the womb.*

> *Do practice this exercise (even just the humming) because deeply focusing on both the sound and vibration can be of great value during your upcoming labor (between contractions, for example). It not only calms the mind but can also help ease pain by giving you something powerfully and actively positive on which to concentrate.*
> *Try just humming a long single note at various times during the day, particularly if you are alone and feeling a little down or have some moments of feeling anxious.*

EXERCISE 25

Letting go the vocalised mantra technique

Although deeply calming and soothing, the chanting of a mantra is still not meditating because your mind remains full of a sound and your attention is on the lulling vibration. When you are ready, you can practice letting go the technique as in the previous exercise.

> *As before, reach into your tension-free body and start slow deep breathing.*
> *Introduce AUM and settle on the chanting of it.*
> *When ready, gradually fade it away to silence, just as you have done with the mind-mantra.*
> *Complete by bringing your awareness back to the gentle rhythm of your breathing.*

Notes:
> *Again, if thoughts start jumping in, simply bring your mantra up in volume to drown them out and then repeat the turning down until you can simply dwell in the silence.*
> *The key to this practice is hushing the voice very gradually. Eventually, there is simply an awareness that you are again being present in silence.*

Quieting technique of focusing on breathing

One of the most popular of the classic techniques practiced for deep mental composure is focusing your awareness single-pointedly on your *hara* breathing and simply staying there, rather than moving on to another technique.

So, in this next exercise, the practice is to just use your breathing as the quieting technique—as the actual point of focus itself.

EXERCISE 26

Breathing as the point of focus

› *Reach your essential stillness to the point of settling into the rhythm of the breathing.*

› *But this time, do not introduce your mantra. Just let your whole mind rest in the deep awareness of the breath coming in and out through your nose and the beautiful rhythm of your slow, gentle, natural breathing.*

› *When thoughts wander in, acknowledge them as the trigger to take your mind-focus back to just sinking into the rhythm of breathing.*

Notes:

› *The aim is to keep your mind on that awareness—focusing single-pointedly on sinking into the harmony created in your body by the gentleness of the rhythm.*

› *Gradually, you will find that focusing on the rhythm creates an increasing intermission between individual thoughts.*

EXERCISE 27

Letting go the breathing technique

Obviously it's not a good idea to let go breathing entirely! Instead, you deepen the practice until you experience a 'oneness' with your breathing, which then enables you to sink into the beautiful stillness of mind, just as you experienced with the vocalised mantra.

› *You are breathing very deeply and slowly, virtually imperceptibly, now.*
› *The next step is to imagine the life-force being breathed in from the universe through every pore of your body—in other words, as if you are breathing through your skin.*
› *Visualize this life-force filling every part of your body with energy and vitality (which is exactly what breathing does).*
› *When breathing out, imagine the reverse. You are breathing out the used-up air back into the universe through every pore of your body.*
› *Maintain deep focus on this imagery until you find you have let go the conscious awareness of deliberately breathing.*
› *To complete, commence with a deep lung-filling breath before moving to your slow movements and so on.*

Notes:
› *If thoughts come in, be aware of them and just keep returning your focus to your breathing.*
› *During this exercise, you will find that gradually you will lose awareness of the boundary of your body. You begin to feel as though life is just coming into you from a vast space. You will begin to have a sense, not of breathing, but of being breathed.*
› *You may begin to lose a sense of yourself as a separate entity and feel as though you are at one with everything as you sink into gentle, aware silence. At that point, the letting go mission will have been accomplished as you dwell in meditation.*

Quieting technique of practicing with open eyes

Many monks of the *Soto Schu* tradition of Zen meditation practice with their eyes open or, what we call, half-lidded or half-open. I include this exercise for you, not just because it is another classic way to quieten the mind, but also for the fact that it is brilliant practice for learning how to maintain intense focus—despite distractions.

For some of you, practicing mind-quieting exercises with your eyes open may initially prove harder than with closed eyes because your vision floods with the distracting images you see before you. For others who find your babbling thoughts intensifying the moment you close your eyes, you may find practicing with opened eyes a revelation (as one student described it to me).

Before going to your sanctuary again, select a small, simple object to take with you—a flower, a leaf, a colored-glass sphere, a little river stone—anything you find lovely and which has a restful color. I often used a clear glass marble. At other times, I used a flower that I had dipped into water, creating crystal-like droplets that clung to it.

EXERCISE 28

Zen practice 1—opening eyes onto an object

> › *Place your object (say, a flower) on the mat before you so that it is in clear focus.*
> › *Commence the practice with closed eyes and proceed to your essential stillness.*
> › *Once settled into your hara or rhythm breathing for five minutes or so, open your eyes, immediately fixing your gaze upon the flower.*
> › *Relax your eyelids so that they are half-open, avoiding a tension-filled, round-eyed staring.*
> › *Continue to hold your gaze on the object. Don't forget to blink.*
> › *If thoughts come to mind, be aware of them and bring your attention back to 'just this flower'.*
> › *Then continue bringing yourself back until you are able to rest in just gazing.*
> › *To complete, close your eyes before returning awareness to your breathing.*

Notes:

› *When you first open your eyes, you may feel a flooding of quite startling visual alertness because of the sudden contrast between your inner awareness and outer seeing.*

› *Gradually, your response will settle as your thoughts begin to wilt under your focused gazing. (One of Suni's other monks once said to me, 'Just stare at the thing until your mind gets bored and shuts up!')*

› *As you will find from practicing other techniques, the space between thoughts will just seem to lengthen as your awareness of the object deepens to fill the mind, leaving less and less space for mental flurry.*

Experiences of a Zen practice

Just as there may be little meditative experiences with your eyes-closed practice, there can be some natural experiences that will occur when just gazing. I mention some of them so you fully understand again that any little experiences are perfectly normal—basically, just simple optical illusions created by an intensity of gazing.

❋ The colors of your object may gradually seem to be so brilliant that it shines or luminesces.

❋ You may begin to see the intricacy of your object's shape, color, texture and lines in a way that you have never seen before. For example, I experienced a powerfully heightened sense of rainbow lights in the water droplets on my flower.

❋ You may have deeper experiences such as the 'vortex sensation' in which the environment in your general peripheral vision around the object becomes a kind of swirling, neutral blur of color with a vortex at the centre in which the flower is in perfect focus. All normal.

❋ You may lose a sense of the distance between you and the object.

- You may also have visions such as seeing auras of different colors around the object but, as with all auras, they are just natural optical illusions.
- You may seem to lose your sense of separateness from your object. In other words, you might lose the sense that you are here and the object is there. You may have the experience of becoming 'one with' the object.

EXERCISE 29

Zen practice 2—complete meditation with open eyes

This next exercise is similar to the previous one, but increases the degree of difficulty because it entails reaching all Essences with your eyes open (half-lidded) from the beginning to the end of the practice. It is one of the most important of the meditative exercises because it can be used as a quite miraculous on-the-run practice for easing tension, anxiety and apprehension. It can also be invaluable for you during your pregnancy, on the way to the birthing place, during labor and delivery and then, if you wish, for the rest of your life.

› *Set your object before you as you did last time and sit in front of it.*
› *Focus your attention on the centre of the object.*
› *Gaze intently at it (you can blink) to minimise external distraction.*
› *When your eyes have settled into gazing, take your mind-awareness inwards and let go tension from your body. Shift it to slow breathing, exactly as you have been practicing, but now with your eyes open.*
› *The next step involves taking your mind-focus outwards as you redirect deep mind-attention to the object on which you have been keeping eye-vigilance.*
› *As you cement your awareness on the object, use it as your single point of focus to quieten your thoughts. Gradually the intensity of your concentrated attention will reduce them to stillness.*
› *Complete when ready (see below).*

Completing a Zen practice with eyes open

The early part of completing a totally eyes-open practice is different to your usual way because, this time, you complete the exercise with eyes open as well.

> *When you feel ready to complete, focus back on your breathing for a while.*
> *Gently look away from the object (say to a general area of the wall or floor).*
> *Begin to slowly move your hands and then the rest of your body, completing as usual.*

Notes:

> *If you find your mind wandering while gazing at the object, just be aware of it and then come back to just gazing.*
> *You can use this lovely practice as an active meditation to settle your mind whenever you have the chance. Anything can be your point of focus, from a spoon on the table to the design on the coffee froth at your favourite coffee house. Try just gazing at the object while letting go tension as you slow and deepen your breathing.*
> *Just three minutes of this lovely practice can be calming and refreshing.*

EXERCISE 30

Letting go the open-eyes technique

The practice now is to use the object you gazed at as the very means of letting go the technique of gazing. You can then drift into stillness, quite unaware of the object and able to dwell in meditative silence.

> *Commence an open-eyes practice with your object placed before you.*
> *As before, stare at your object until you quieten your body, breathing and thoughts.*

The aim now is to move from staring intently at the object to the act of gazing through it until you reach awareness without seeing.

› *To do this, you gradually shift your focus to a point on the other side of the object. That point can be a metre past it or somewhere on the other side of the universe.*

› *You are simply moving your point of focus so that you are gazing through your object to that distant point.*

› *Just rest in the peacefulness of gazing.*

› *When you are ready to complete, slowly direct your focus back onto the physical object before you.*

› *After a little while, bring your mind-awareness back to your breathing and settle it there before completing in the usual way.*

› *Take your time so that the calmness carries with you into your day.*

Notes:

› *If you settle into this practice for long enough, sometimes just 10 or so minutes, you will find that the object completely disappears. Of course, in reality it doesn't. It's just that gazing through the object gently takes you to your inner peaceful awareness where you become present and dwell, rather than paying attention to the object.*

› *In this exercise, prior to actually experiencing that deep inner stillness, you may well have some further visual experiences. You may see that your object is out of focus and, accordingly, an array of visual effects and optical illusions may occur. Any experience is harmless and natural and will gradually pass as your practice deepens. Any such experience is again simply a little signpost that you are indeed mastering your ability to focus intently and quieten your busy mind . . . wonderful for later on.*

› *It is a beautiful practice to take with you anywhere. Try practicing in a garden of flowers or on the beach.*

The beginning of genuine meditation

In practicing letting go any of the techniques to quieten the mind's constant prattle, you soon reach a stage on this peaceful journey when you begin to just sink into a supreme mental quietness. This is the beginning of true meditation—just dwelling in peacefulness.

It is a beautiful soul-garden place, devoid of all the usual distractions of tension, unmastered thought, needless mental conditioning and wobbling emotions. When you are fully present in the quietness, you are naturally unencumbered by any pressures, the stress of expectations or tormenting negative emotions. There is no annoyance, anger, sadness or grief. There is no sense of anxiety, fear or feelings of depression, all of which are felt in the normal life as suffering or unhappiness. Conversely, nor are you burdened by transient extremes of self-satisfaction, excitement, over-exuberance or excessive zeal—the illusions often mistaken for happiness.

Now this doesn't mean we become non-thinking, non-feeling, non-emotional automatons. In fact, authentic meditation has the absolute reverse effect. It lets us back in to access who we really are. Without a busy mind, the uncluttered consciousness we experience becomes a clear space in which our human potency, our original perceptive magnificence and loving compassion are able to reawaken or resurface.

By genuinely practicing meditating in a state of quiet peacefulness, you can also re-equip yourself with a compelling strength of mind, a well of inner energy and an intensity of will, all quite undiluted and priceless in times of apprehension, pain and extreme exertion. This is the greatest gift you can give yourself if you are trying to become a mom, an actual mom-to-be or a new mom.

Danielle's story

Little Evangeline Rose

About eight months ago, you kindly shared your 'Meditation-during-Pregnancy' information with me. I had experienced a very painful labor first time around and was looking to make the second much better.

I was only ever a meditation beginner but I tried to practice daily when putting our first child to sleep each night. As the second pregnancy neared its end, I was sure I was not ready for the labor as I hadn't been as committed, as I had hoped, to my meditation practice.

Unfortunately I again had to be induced (flashes of horror from labor number one) but that's where the comparisons ended.

This time, it was a painful but peaceful labor and I can only credit the meditation practice. Although I had to be monitored and confined to the bed, I didn't take any gas or drugs and breathed through the pain. Evangeline Rose was born after almost five hours of labor, three pushes and no stitches.

Evie has just turned nine months and is a delight.

I'm so pleased to see that your book on meditation for motherhood is being published. I can only recommend the practice!

CHAPTER SEVEN

Mindfulness: the art of focusing on 'just this', 'just now'

*I've sat and watched the giant tree in the drive shed its
leaves in showers of confetti on the wind. Perhaps, more
importantly, I've just sat . . .*

WENDY LIMOND—SANCTUARY STUDENT

Mindfulness is the ability to not just be present in the moment but
be wholly awake to experiencing each moment of life with crystal-
clear consciousness. It is the meditative art of letting go the mental
load of conditioned thoughts, behaviour, attitudes and judgements
that burden most people. In other words, it is a state of transparent
awakeness that leaves us open to seeing and focusing purely on 'just
this', 'just now'. When we are perfectly present, attending the 'now',
we are again deeply and single-pointedly focused on each moment

of living just as small children and all animals are naturally—the whole time. A wonderful woman and Zen monk, Geri Larkin, says in her book, *Stumbling Towards Enlightenment*:

> . . . *the practice of mindfulness means . . . not missing a moment of this extraordinary journey which is your life. Even the smallest segment can teach you unfathomable lessons—not to mention the peace, understanding and even joy in the face of all the storms that come our way.*[1]

With practice, mindfulness means being truly conscious of our senses, thoughts (and attached emotions), our self and our behaviour. In this chapter, we are going to look at simple practices of becoming mindful of those aspects of life so you can apply this valuable second stream of meditation to just about every situation you face and manage them with increasing composure and poise.

Mindfulness of our senses

Be honest now. Do you remember feeling the soothing water warming your body in the shower this morning? Or were you so busy thinking about the worries of the day ahead that you were barely aware of even being in the shower? Did you offer a goodbye kiss that gave nourishment to your heart-love for the day, or was it just a habit-filled, busy-person peck.

It is a truth that most people are so brain-occupied that they actually perceive 10 percent or less of the available life-information available to them through their senses moment by moment— about themselves, their various relationships, life in general or the lovely universe of which they happen to be a part. I often say that people are 90 percent asleep most of the time because they are too busy thinking and worrying—in other words, living life in their head rather than fully experiencing it moment by precious moment.

The senses of genuinely meditative people, on the other hand, are finely tuned to be 100 percent awake. When they see, they see everything because they are not looking through a warping veil of conditioned thought that lies between what they think they see and what really is—unlike most people. When they listen, they really hear each wave of sound. When they eat, they eat slowly and taste each morsel with thankful joy. When they smell, it is with an aware pleasure that they can. When they touch an object or a person, each time it is as if for the first time.

Quite simply, their core faculties are all open at the same time. They tend to be in a natural state of pure, sensory mindfulness. It is like having a sixth sense.

It is quite simple. If we are really tasting and enjoying that morsel with awareness, we are not lost in thought and negative emotions. If we are smiling at a willie-wagtail's antics, we cannot be filled with dread or anxiety. We are busy being occupied with just this, just now. It is logical that the more we can practice 'being here', the less we allow the debris of worry to become a burden. Go watch a small child at play. See how her entire sensory being is fully awake in this moment. Mindfulness is the way to unexpected moments of joy and longer times of balanced peacefulness.

EXERCISE 31

Just listening—the practice template for all the senses

If I asked you to write down all the sounds you remember having heard in the past half hour, without stopping and listening, you would actually list very few—probably not more than two or three. If you really listen, however, you will hear 20 or 30 sounds in just a few minutes, all which were there, but you were too busy thinking to hear them. Surprise yourself with this treasure of an exercise in mindfulness.

> Sit anywhere, inside or outdoors, close your eyes and really listen. Then write down every sound you can hear for about 10 to 15 minutes.

> Try now to become single-pointedly aware of just listening—really giving mind-focused attention to identifying sounds.

> When you finish, try and recall what you felt when you were just listening.

You will soon realize that the world out there is abuzz with sound, as if the whole universe is resonating with noise. For a few minutes, you were actually mindful—you just listened!

In writing down the sounds you heard, however, you were still having some thoughts because you identified each sound with a name and labelled it. The meditative endevor is to let go any response at all—in other words, to just listen, not just with your ears but with your entire being, without thought. That is perfect mindfulness.

EXERCISE 32

Listening without a conditioned response

Select a beautiful piece of music. (For this exercise in class, I often use Mozart's *Concerto in C* or sometimes a recording of bird sounds.)

> Start the music when you are ready and then reach your essential stillness.

> Take your awareness to your listening, but this time just immerse yourself in the sound, trying not to think about what you are hearing.

> Open yourself to the sound as a small child listens when she doesn't yet know the words to interpret the sounds. Listen with your whole body.

> If thoughts intrude, just use the music as your point of focus until the thoughts fade.

> Complete when you are ready.

After a while, you will begin to experience the feeling of 'oneness with the music'—with the sound. You will feel that you are the sound. That is mindful listening—being perfectly present because you have removed the senses-numbing veil of conditioned thinking.

Again, you can practice this second stream of meditation, mindfulness or awakeness whenever you wish, wherever you go. Just stop and pay attention. Gradually you will find that you change from just hearing sound to really listening to sound.

The remaining senses—finding miracles

I could go through all the senses with exercises for each one but they are effectively identical. The mastery of deep focusing is to simply and consciously pay attention to just being in every moment with each of your senses. It sounds easy to 'just be' but it does take a little effort because we get so easily sidetracked and distracted by our non-stop thoughts. So becoming really mindful is not an overnight miracle.

Given that mindfulness is natural, however, it still rests within every human being and can be reached into just by daring to try. Deliberately allocate some time each day to stop, rest awhile, then really just listen, see, smell, taste and touch until eventually, you can do it again naturally, just as you did as a small child.

Slowly, and with a sense of wonderment, you realize that it is much easier to just be 'here' focusing on 'this' rather than sitting with your mind in top gear, getting sick with worry and agitation. I called the reawakening of our senses 'finding miracles', because that is exactly what it feels like.

Mindfulness of thinking

Layering on the mindfulness of thinking, which I also call nourished or intentional thinking, can further enhance your experience of waking up to the vibrancy of life.

It is our thinking alone that clouds our focus and burdens us with unwanted, unnecessary worries. But our thoughts and the ensuing emotions needn't be driven along mindlessly like tumbleweed in the wind. There is another way.

With even just a little practice, it is possible for the meditating person to enhance his or her calmness and life efficiency by developing a meditative way of thinking. This means choosing when you want to think, what you want to think about and, most importantly, being able to stay focused on a subject without being distracted from it.

EXERCISE 33

Focused thinking

The first step towards becoming more genuinely in control of your mind is not only being aware of what you are thinking, but keeping yourself on a chosen thought-track without getting snatched away by associated thoughts in which you soon get lost.

› *Begin by asking yourself, 'What am I thinking right now?'*
› *Try and watch your thoughts and be aware when the subject changes.*
› *When you notice that you are off-track, bring your mind back to the first thought-subject. Try to hold onto it for a little longer before wandering away again.*
› *Repeat this several times, always bringing yourself back to 'just this'.*

EXERCISE 34

Nourished thinking, nourished emotions

The benefits of being able to confine ourselves to what we want to think about are immeasurable. As I have said, the main one is that it stops our emotions being dragged uncontrollably from pillar to post, which happens because our emotions are hopelessly entwined with our thoughts.

> *After some days of practicing the previous exercise, close your eyes and begin to ask yourself another question: 'What, ideally, could I be thinking about right now that could be more positive and helpful to my day, this week or my life?'*
> *When you have chosen a subject, try really hard to stay with that subject and contemplate it single-pointedly.*
> *When you notice that you have wandered, that is fine. Just gently remind yourself of the subject and bring yourself back to it again.*

Quieting emotions

This doesn't require much extra effort because steadiness of emotions is a natural, virtually automatic result of balanced, nourished thinking. So, in being more mindful through calm, focused thinking, it is possible to be emotionally more balanced, even under physical duress.

With practice, you can also begin to direct your thoughts more consciously and beneficially in order to have a calming effect on your emotions—a greatly beneficial skill to have throughout your pregnancy and then delivery.

> *After you have become more adept at staying with a subject, begin to notice what you are feeling while contemplating the subject.*
> *Whether a positive or negative emotion, just bring yourself back to focusing deeply on the subject until the emotion quietly fades.*
> *Complete this exercise by changing your mind-awareness away from the subject to your slow deep breathing (giving your mind a little rest).*

Notes:
> *Do practice this exercise as often as you can. It is not difficult because it is simply an extension of your practicing the single-minded focus you gave to other exercises such as letting go thoughts or listening with your whole being.*

> *Importantly, try practicing this as you go about your daily life. Focus your mind increasingly on the business at hand, from washing the dishes to planning a holiday next year. Try to be aware of wandering so you can bring yourself back to 'just this'.*

> *Practicing being awake strengthens confidence in trusting your own wisdom as you increasingly perceive harmful negative thoughts and self-attitude and then being able to let them go using your mindfulness techniques.*

Self-awareness

A very simple way to check on your emotional state of mind throughout your pregnancy is to actually pay attention to your speech. Being mindful of the way you speak and what you actually say is like holding up a mirror to see a reflection of your thinking and emotions.

EXERCISE 35

Mindfully listening to yourself—another way to calmness

How you speak

> *Whenever you remember, try and listen to yourself speaking, just as if you were listening to someone else.*

> *Try and notice the difference in the speech modes of people with whom you converse.*

> *Endevor to perceive any correlation between the way you speak and your emotional state at the time.*

Notes:

> *You will soon see that a person who speaks gently and slowly also appears to be calm. Then quite the opposite, a harsh, loud and grating voice is a sure sign of someone who is internally agitated in some way.*

> *The message is clear. Endevoring to speak slowly and in a more*

peaceful way is another meditative tool to let go stress in a tense situation.

› *Speaking slowly and gently is a wonderful practice to work on before the little one is born because your soothing, calm voice, reflecting an inner peacefulness, is like a neon sign on a hill to a baby: 'Mom is calm—all is well with my world.'*

What you say

Being mindful of the manner and content of your speech is another way you can prevent spilling your calmness.

› *Begin listening to what you say.*

› *What emotions were you expressing while speaking?*

› *Note whether it was important or was babble.*

› *Do you think it mattered to anyone other than you?*

Notes:

› *The meditative person tries to be mindful of what he or she says. I once wrote, 'Harm no other with your voice or the content of your talking. Mindfully practice every aspect of your speaking. You have ample opportunity . . . as in every single time you open your mouth to utter a sound.'*

› *I tell my students that if you have nothing positive, emotionally or spiritually nutritious to say, then say nothing. The meditative person never babbles for attention. Use quietness to enhance your inner peacefulness.*

Mindfulness of actions

Most people are in a perpetual state of rushing. They move hastily, clumsily, thoughtlessly. They can be uncoordinated and unattractive in their physical actions. But they don't mean to be this way. They are just all full of tension from stress that unconsciously affects the very way they physically move.

The ideal way is exactly the opposite. The way you physically move is another path to self-observation because the actions of your body (just like your speech) are also a mirror-perfect reflection of your state of mind. The key to mindfulness of action and activities is quite simple—slow down!

EXERCISE 36

Calmness through mindfulness of actions

› As you are going about your daily busyness, begin to notice how you actually move.

› When you notice that you too have a stiffness or rushed jerkiness in your actions, begin to practice moving with peaceful deliberateness and gracefulness—physical mindfulness.

› Practice doing everything a little more slowly.

› Try to be deliberate rather than doing things in a mundane, bored or automatic way.

Notes:

› By being mindfully deliberate and gracefully conservative with your body and your energy, you will increasingly find that, with less effort, you seem to be doing much more. This is because, by slowing down, you actually give attention to everything you do. This eliminates all the time wasted when our minds and bodies are used ineffectively— when they are flurried and worried.

› The meditative person begins to give full, mindful attention to every second of life so that gradually, all action is deeply experienced because it has deliberate and joyful purpose in the doing of anything and everything.

EXERCISE 37

Calmness through mindfulness of behaviour

A consistent attempt to behave as an awakening being means that we realize that every moment of our life is for practicing the way we treat ourselves and the way we behave towards others. It begins to give us a peacefulness brought on by mindfully offering the best of ourselves with kindness, love and compassion.

When you become a new mother, you have in your arms one of the perfect ways to practice this highest level of mindfulness. To unfold a deeper peacefulness throughout pregnancy and afterwards, you may like to try some of these meditative practices.

› *Be kind to everyone—with no motive—even if that is just a smile at a stranger.*
› *Never say or repeat anything hurtfully negative about another.*
› *Meditate on difficulties. Listen to your inner being for wisdom.*
› *Don't punish yourself. If the plate is broken, it is broken. That is one of the great awakenings, realising what is. Move on.*
› *Be honest in what you say and do. Hurt no other being with your words or deeds.*
› *Give openly of yourself without needing reward or recognition.*
› *Practice appreciating and enjoying the lightness of just being.*

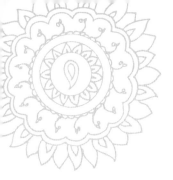

CHAPTER EIGHT

Visualization: the benefits of focused imagination

As I outlined earlier, we spend quite a lot of thinking time in the future. When thinking about the future—either daydreaming or wishful thinking—we use our imagination, much of which is based on our memory of a similar experience. We create little mind plays, with our self as the central character. The amazing thing is that in creating images about something in the future, such as giving birth, you have an emotional response as if the event were actually happening to you at this moment. Conversely, imagining our visit to the dentist tomorrow can make us feel queasy in the stomach, right now.

So, it is our busy, batty brain that causes us to be happy or unhappy when we are imagining events in a future that is not here yet—and we do this constantly.

Mastering imagination

Just as we can meditatively focus our thoughts for emotional benefit, so too we can harness our imagination in a practice called creative visualization. This can be of considerable benefit not only to our emotional stability but to our entire wellbeing.

By learning to turn daydreaming, fantasising and wishful thinking (all our crazy little mind plays) into creative visualization, we can develop another powerful meditative life-tool, just like letting go tension, natural breathing and quieting the mind. Visualization can be applied to many aspects of our life, from changing negative behavioural patterns to considering future events with emotional clearness and maturity rather than with apprehension.

Above all for moms-to-be, you can use visualization while meditating in such a way that you can experience the possibilities of a future event and train yourself in advance to manage them—and your emotions—in a positive way. While making visualization work for you effectively can take a little time, it is a great way of being emotionally prepared for labor and birth, rather than experiencing alarm over unexpected events or surprises on this special journey.

EXERCISE 38

Remembering—the starting point of imagination

You will need your writing book and pen.

> *Think of the most beautiful place that you have been or seen.*
> *Close your eyes and imagine you are there for a little while. Remember as many details of your lovely place as you can.*
> *Now write down as many little particulars as possible, such as how your special place smells, sounds, looks like, what features stand out, what the temperature is and so on.*

Notes:
> *Make your beautiful place one in which you could rest happily, by yourself, for hours at a time.*

> *In our class practice we call this 'being in your inner sanctuary', because in times of stress, you can find peace by visiting your special place whenever you wish.*

EXERCISE 39

Meditating in your inner sanctuary—creative visualization

> *Start your normal meditation by moving through the Three Essences and rest in stillness for a few minutes.*
> *When you are ready, bring to mind (visualize) your special place.*
> *With closed eyes, sit in it, feel it, smell it, hear it, look around and enjoy it.*
> *Be aware of the peacefulness and dwell in that tranquillity.*
> *Gradually let the sanctuary fade by taking your awareness back to your breathing and complete.*

Note:
> *In this exercise, you will move from remembering details of your inner sanctuary to actually experiencing it as if you were there—that is visualization.*
> *Visualization is far more effective if you dwell in meditation first. When you are quiet of mind, you have created a perfectly clear space within, so anything you visualize will have much greater clarity.*

Using visualization to overcome difficulties

After becoming adept at the last exercise, creative visualization can be applied widely to provide greater insight and clarity on many aspects of our being. There are countless examples of this lovely meditative practice having a positive effect on people's lives.

In our own Meditation Sanctuary, I have witnessed the benefits experienced by so many students over the years. Some have given up smoking or drinking or drugs or other obsessive behaviours by practicing visualizing their lives without these negative escape routes from suffering. Many have overcome debilitating anxiety and depression—permanently—through a balanced practice of meditation and visualization.

The lovely thing is visualization is so accessible and can be used by any meditating person to overcome difficulties or enhance life in some way. It can be used for everything from simply visualizing yourself as a calm person, being calm at the dentist, completing a project, improving your work attitude and quality of work, being successful at something, enhancing sporting performance, mending relationships and even having a more peaceful birth (we'll get to that soon).

EXERCISE 40

Putting visualization to work

For this exercise, select an area of your life or an issue in which you would ideally like to see some positive change. I shall use the example of improving a relationship when there has been argument (that should cover just about everybody!). Remember, these are training exercises and you can, of course, choose any situation you wish.

› *Begin your normal meditation by moving through the Three Essences and then rest in stillness.*

› *When you are ready, recall and review a recent argument, but try not to be emotionally responsive in your remembering—just recall.*

› *After reviewing it as it was, visualize the situation again but, this time, act out in your mind how it could have been or how you would have preferred it to be. For example, instead of speaking a harsh word, visualize speaking a word of kindness or not responding to harshness.*

› *Instead of, say, walking out in anger, visualize offering a cup of tea or putting out a hand towards the other in a gesture of warmth and goodwill.*

› *Stay with the visualization, recreating the situation until you are ready to complete.*
› *Repeat this practice as often as you wish.*

Notes:

› *When you become more accomplished at sinking easily into visualization meditations, you may be astonished to find yourself responding to issues in your life in a much wiser and warmer manner. Redirecting your behaviour towards the positive can also have a remarkable effect on others.*

› *The great lesson of visualization is that we increasingly see and understand that issues, worries and apprehensions need not be a natural part of our life. They are essentially 'out there', not 'in here', and envisaging a more ideal or positive outcome can radically alter our responses from negative to increasingly positive.*

› *For the seriously meditative person, his or her entire life can slowly begin to transcend the petty, shallow, uptight, tension-filled and self-centred way of being that, ultimately, is the most stressful way of living. Even expressing just one of those traits can have an effect on the baby's emotional status. Meditation, with a layer of visualization when needed, can be a life-changer, even for the unborn.*

Using visualization to renew wellbeing

I will not tell you that meditation and visualization can heal you, but there is a wealth of international research demonstrating that practicing these two natural skills can have a profound effect on our total wellbeing, including our physical wellbeing. So if you are experiencing any unwellness, including morning sickness, you might like to practice this exercise.

EXERCISE 41

Wellbeing visualization

› *Move through the Three Essences and dwell in the stillness for a little while.*

› *When you are ready, visualize the air you breathe in as a golden, health-giving life-force.*

› *With each in-breath imagine healthy life filling your lungs, overflowing into every cell of your body.*

› *As you breathe out, visualize the color being breathed out and being renewed. Do this for several minutes.*

› *Take your inner awareness and focus to the area affected by physical (or even mental or emotional) difficulty.*

› *Now visualize wrapping the area of illness in a blanket of golden, light-filled life-energy that you draw from the air into your body.*

› *Visualize breathing out that golden cloud, pushing it out into space with your breath, along with the sickness it is wrapped around, and watch it fade away.*

› *Tell it to go. Watch it go. Believe it is going. Know it is going.*

› *Repeat this exercise over and over.*

› *Return to just meditating, dwelling within the serene space before completing.*

Note:

› *Remember, this is a technique, not a cure, but it is one that can have quite an extraordinary effect because it brings into full play the deeply powerful and natural resources of your own mind.*

Visualizing through the birth phases

It is possible to practice visualizing the various stages of labor and birth from beginning to end. There are two key potential benefits of practicing these visualizations. Firstly, you can visualize yourself remaining calm through the difficult stages. Secondly, you can reduce apprehension and anxiety about, for example, anticipated pain and weariness by being prepared for them through having already 'experienced' them within the quietness of a meditative context.

Before you begin, if you decide to include these helpful exercises, become really familiar with the various phases of late-stage pregnancy—your waters breaking, labor and the birthing process. Consult trusted others or professionals such as your doctor or a midwife. You may wish to watch videos, but make sure they are of the highest, professional quality in their knowledge and advice such as the beautiful, brilliant and moving *The Odyssey of Life*[2] series.

I have also outlined the three stages of labor and delivery in Chapter 14 and offer suggestions on which practices apply to help you through each of those phases.

But know that your own journey is, and will continue to be, unique to you. No book, article, person or video can describe or forecast your particular experience. But the phases of becoming a mother are essentially common to all and you can be better prepared by becoming more familiar with them in your visualization practice.

Then later, when you are actually experiencing them, you may have the comfort of saying to yourself, 'Okay, I know where I'm up to right now. I can use the right meditative practice to give me a hand.'

EXERCISE 42

Late-stage visualizations

Before you start any of these practices, choose just one aspect of the late-stage journey to be visualized within each meditation.

The following exercise only uses one phase (early contractions) as an example, but as you progress, simply replace the last phase in your meditative visualization with the next one.

> Start your normal meditation by moving through the Three Essences. This is especially important now.

> Let go the technique (mantra, for example) you have used for achieving single-pointed focus and dwell in the stillness for a little while.

> Slowly begin to visualize an early contraction (for example). As it tightens and begins to be painful, feel it in your mind.

> As you experience the imagined pain of tightening, deliberately focus on the calmness of your breathing. Try and let go tension in your whole belly area.

> Focus on the visualized contraction subsiding and the pain easing. Then move your mind-focus to letting go tension again and breathing gently.

> Endevor to include in your visualization little moments (even if tiny) of a sense of joy at the true wonderment of what you are and will be doing.

Notes:

> Do not try these visualizations until you have spent at least a month or two (at least once a week) honing your visualization skills on the earlier exercises.

> It is an absolute key to potential benefits that you only practice the birth visualizations after you really have reached your essential stillness each time—being deeply tension-free, slow and deep of breathing and quiet of mind. Always start with this natural preparation as you have been doing for all exercises.

> In the practice and later, in reality, you may feel that it is difficult or even silly to try and let go tension and be calm when you are in the throes of a painful contraction or during delivery. Of course it can be difficult but, with practice, it is possible and potentially highly beneficial if you can master these skills.

> Pain of contractions and delivery is quite unlike other pain (such as cutting yourself) but nevertheless, similarly affects your whole body. It shallows the breathing, increases body tension, increases the heart rate and raises blood pressure—all of which can amplify the pain. Logically then, if you can bring yourself to greater calmness during the painful times, the above effects can be somewhat diminished.

> Quite simply, if you focus on your breathing and let go tension, you can relieve pain to a lesser or greater extent. With due practice, the calmer you are, the lighter the pain you may suffer and the more focused you are, the less apprehension you may experience.

EXERCISE 43

Smiling meditation

This is a miscellaneous little meditation that you can do wherever you are at any time. It is very effective because it releases oxytocins (a 'feel-good' hormone) from the brain, which enhances your sense of wellbeing. This can be one of your lovely, anti-apprehension weapons along the way.

> Reach your stillness.
> Before dwelling in your serene space, imagine yourself smiling. Feel yourself smiling, but not with your mouth which remains as still as you can keep it.
> Smile with your whole body—your eyes, your face, your tummy, your hands etc.
> Complete, but take the warm feeling with you when you go about your day.

The main message of Part One is that the practice of meditation and visualization during your pregnancy, as a minimum, will give you delightful moments of true rest, calmness and peace. These skills potentially offer you the most positive benefits all the way to holding your beautiful baby joyfully in your arms.

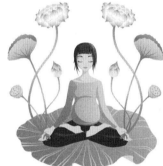

PART TWO

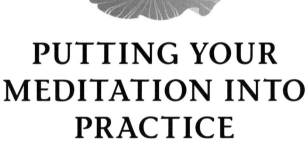

PUTTING YOUR MEDITATION INTO PRACTICE

CHAPTER NINE

Meditation for conception: health, stress and fertility

Worldwide scientific research on foetal development has now proven beyond doubt that the mother's approach to her own health and mental wellbeing, from the moment her egg is fertilised, has a profound and probably life-long effect on the wellbeing of her child. Accordingly, I recommend that, from the very moment you start on your motherhood mission, your first commitment is to commence meditation while also taking on board the common-sense health and lifestyle suggestions in this chapter.

Starting meditation at the true beginning of your journey gives you an extraordinary advantage because, by the time you are ready to give birth, you will have developed a sound knowledge of how and when to maximize the benefits of meditation at all phases of your pregnancy and beyond.

For about one in six couples, however, the joyful decision to make a baby can become a year or more of gradually sinking hearts and a slowly rising anxiety as—nothing happens. There can be a dawning realization that, as a couple, you may be infertile, either for no apparent reason or because of a known difficulty.

In this chapter, then, I will discuss the suspects known to cause difficulties becoming pregnant and some proactive steps you can take to combat them. I will then look at the key issue of whether stress can cause infertility as well as reduce the potential success of IVF treatment and show how meditation is becoming a potent tool in overcoming such specific difficulties.

Overall, though, the essential focus of the chapter is to illustrate that the practice of meditation, in enhancing total-life health and wellbeing, is today proving to be a mainstream method in the medical world of increasing the possibility of success in both spontaneous and assisted pregnancy.

Health and fertility

A well-known Australia medical practitioner, Dr Sandra Cabot, in her excellent book *Infertility: The Hidden Cause*[3] has used the phrase 'a healthy body is a fertile body'. Many other researchers have reinforced the fact that a deficiency in general health, so often caused by stress, can be a key factor in temporary or unexplained infertility. But couples can do much to increase their chances of becoming pregnant naturally. It is possible to improve fertility with a sensible, positive and enjoyable wellness program—for both women and men. (Men are actually responsible for around 40 percent of infertility due to low or very low sperm count[4] but this can, in some instances, be reversed with an increase in general health.)

Overcoming physical problems preventing pregnancy

There is a range of physical issues that, with appropriate treatment and attention, can enhance your chances of having a baby, even if you have been experiencing difficulties.

Infections

These can include, for example, genital infections in both men and women, pelvic infections, blocked fallopian tubes, ovarian cysts, endometriosis and PCOS (polycystic ovarian syndrome). If you are having difficulty getting pregnant, the first step for both of you is to visit your doctor for a check-up because most infections can now be treated effectively.

Overweight

Numerous researchers suggest that being overweight is the most important factor in temporary infertility and can be a pronounced factor in less successful IVF treatments. A key, common-sense factor in restoring fertility is losing weight through regular exercise and right nutrition. Any form of exercise such as walking, swimming, yoga (more on this later), gardening or cycling, if undertaken daily, will help you lose weight. You can exercise quite vigorously until you're about five months pregnant before slowly tapering off, although walking and gentle forms of yoga can be practiced until full term.

Poor nutrition

The consumption of highly processed foodstuff, if coupled with a lack of fresh fruits and vegetables, is a potent recipe for fertility issues. There is only one approach to getting the right nutrition for your body and that is to eat nutritious food—kind of logical really. Use common sense and perhaps seek out expert nutritional advice such as the 'Fertility Diet' in Dr Cabot's book *Infertility: The Hidden Cause*.

Lack of water—too much alcohol

Most people are unaware of the importance of drinking water. It is a fact, though, that not drinking enough water can cause memory loss, dizziness, kidney dysfunction, intestinal and elimination problems and poor, parched skin. Our bodies are mainly made up of water and it is an essential ingredient for radiant health and a key food for a healthy brain. I consider it as important as breathing. I teach the ancient Zen wisdom that the right daily intake is about eight glasses a day for women and 12 for men.

There is overwhelming evidence to suggest that drinking alcohol can have an inhibiting effect on fertility, particularly in men who drink to excess. Alcohol also has a potentially disastrous effect on an embryo and, later, the fetus.

Renowned French pediatrician, the late Dr Maurice Titran[5] said repeatedly in interviews that alcohol leads to malnutrition and anoxia (lack of oxygen) in the baby. In small doses, alcohol slows down the movement of embryonic and foetal cells. In strong doses it makes them explode. This wise man dubbed abstinence at this time as 'the no-risk level of alcohol consumption'.

Chemical exposure

Chemicals are embedded in just about everything we eat, touch, breathe in, wear, wash with, sit on, lie on, eat, store our food in, spray and adorn ourselves with—the list is frighteningly comprehensive. They are virtually inescapable unless you find a monastery high on a forested mountain near a crystal-clear stream. Scientists worldwide are now saying that being exposed to toxic chemicals is one of the greatest challenges to modern human health.

Again, the only reasonable approach is to find common-sense ways to minimise your exposure. Very good information is readily available on the household chemicals contained in so many products and how you can find sensible, organic alternatives—including food.

Substance intake

In our fast-moving, neurotic society, so many people are resorting to taking substances of one kind or another to pep them up, calm them down or just 'fix' them. Most are relatively harmless in moderation over a short period but all can have a negative effect if you are seeking a refined level of health to enhance fertility. For example, coffee and caffeine-laced energy drinks as well as sugar-filled beverages can cause heart palpitations and physical tension. (Later, I will discuss how tension is one of the great impediments to health and wellbeing.) It is best to moderate or limit your intake of these on your motherhood journey.

Prescription drugs, by their very nature, are poisons. Of course, prescribed wisely, drugs can be of tremendous benefit. But, as a society, we are taking nerve-calmers, sleep-helpers and sickness-fixers at an addictive rate. Check out the possible conception-inhibiting factors of your medications with your doctor.

The nicotine in cigarettes is said to be the most addictive drug of all. If wanting to enhance your fertility, know that smoking is the most serious of chemical exposures. Prenatal researcher Benoist Schaal[6] says that 'the transfer between the mother and her child . . . of medicinal substances and addictive drugs . . . is extremely rapid. Smoking can have a devastating effect on your baby . . . it is at risk of being born underweight or too early.' To have a healthy baby, there is only one solution. Stop poisoning yourself and quit.

Age

After the age of about 35, it becomes more difficult to become pregnant, although it is actually possible up to menopause. There can also be a slightly increased possibility of abnormalities in the fetus carried by an older woman but, encouragingly, the vast majority of children born to women over 35 are perfectly normal. The fertility of men is also affected by age. Men are able to produce sperm into quite advanced years, although the number and motility of them reduces as the decades pass. But, as one wise woman, my editor Katie Stackhouse, said, 'Of course, age can't be changed—all you can do is improve everything else.'

Other health hints

I recently discovered an old book, *Yoga for Women* by Nancy Phelan and Michael Volin, published back in 1963. In a chapter titled 'Sterility', their opening paragraph was intriguing: 'The practice of yoga has so often had beneficial effects on sterile couples that women sometimes say facetiously that they fear to take it up lest they become pregnant.'

Today, classes on yoga for pregnant women are commonplace as the immense benefits of practicing de-stressing and wellbeing are now being widely recognised, particularly by the medical field. I strongly recommend adding gentle *hatha* yoga to your health regimen because it has such a positive effect on the suppleness of the spine and joints, stimulation of the glands (including reproductive), and on the efficient functioning of all your internal systems.

Lifestyle changes

Lifestyle habits can also have an effect on fertility. Develop healthy habits such as getting sufficient sleep, walking in the sun for a daily dose of vitamin D and just resting for body renewal, for which your early meditation exercises will prove invaluable.

I tell my students that the key activity for wellbeing is simply to have fun. Treat yourself from time to time: enjoy friends, love widely and well, rejoice in simple things and laugh a lot. That always makes you feel good. Enjoy the good news of others; be part of the good news of others by finding the time to help or care for others, or even just show kindness to a stranger. This is all wonderful for inner peacefulness—a great place bodies like to be to facilitate conception.

Lovemaking—not just baby-making

Having made the decision to become pregnant, let go the idea of making love for the specific purpose of becoming pregnant. Enjoy your closeness. Revel in just sharing love with your partner—one of the most important reasons for living. This brings in the idea of 'falling pregnant' (just as you 'fell in love'), rather than struggling stressfully to become pregnant. This is a highly meditative idea—doing something for the sake of doing it—rather than trying for a result. Let this baby-making be a spontaneous delight as I believe that joy in lovemaking enhances fertility.

Summary of health and infertility

Perhaps the most compelling reason to give attention to your physical and mental wellbeing before pregnancy is the evidence in a major study relating to health and infertility by experts from the University of Adelaide in South Australia.[7] They reviewed more than 130 clinical studies worldwide on whether lifestyle factors impact on reproductive performance (as well as people undergoing assisted reproductive treatment). They trawled the latest global research on whether such factors as 'age, smoking, weight, diet, exercise, psychological stress, caffeine consumption, alcohol intake and exposure to environmental pollutants are influential in infertility.'

They found comprehensive evidence in these studies that age, weight and smoking impact adversely on general health and reproductive performance. There was further strong indication that all the other lifestyle factors also play a significant part in infertility.

So, if you intend to have a baby, or are having trouble in becoming pregnant, there's so much evidence to support a committed health effort as a sensible starting point. The very worst that can happen is that you are both going to be healthier. Happily, if you add meditation to your health program, you will find that it is not all a new unwelcome chore but a life-refreshing venture.

Selena's story

Keeping active

The key to a good pregnancy, labor and delivery for me was keeping active. In a way, you could say I did a bit of this and a bit of that, but it all helped. I started off doing some prenatal yoga, which a number of hospitals make available. Certainly there are many classes out there for pregnant women and one or two have started up for small children as well.

I mainly did walking, which is great exercise. It can get a little uncomfortable to walk in the later stages but it's still great for you and can help bring on labor towards the end of your time. I also did swimming, which I found just great for pregnancy, and attended an aqua-aerobics class. If they don't have one available specifically for pregnant women, do what I did. I joined the seniors class—the old ladies were just lovely to me!

If you feel you need treatment, I recommend acupuncture and osteopathy. I experienced really severe morning sickness and found that acupuncture helped a lot. Osteopathy was a very holistic approach.

Definitely meditate. In the later stages, I found it uncomfortable so changed to a number of enjoyable five-minute sessions instead of a long 20–30 minute practice.

To sum up, the fitter you are the easier the labor and birth will be. I managed fine although my labor was long and the delivery was also 90 minutes, but I managed the pain without a problem and with no drugs!

Stress—a cause of infertility?

On the morning of my starting this chapter, I caught an inspiring breakfast interview with a happy couple on national television.[8] They unfolded the most heart-warming and extraordinary story of their endeavors to conceive. The woman had experienced 16 IVF treatments (that is not a printing error) resulting in six pregnancies, all of them unsuccessful. In stressed-out desperation, they had advertised several times for a donor egg. Finally, a kind person had made the offer of an egg. The man and the woman said they had been 'over the moon' to have been granted this final opportunity to have a baby.

Before the egg could be harvested, however, the woman becamepregnant naturally, a happy event which the couple had not been able to achieve previously. At the time of interview she was four months pregnant, further than she had been with IVF, and all was well.

Clearly, after such a long and futile journey, both parents-in-hope had become deeply stressed. On just being offered the wonderful gift of a donor egg, however, the stress burden was lifted from their shoulders. With the stress gone, they fell pregnant.

Infertility for no apparent reason

There are many stories of women who finally accepted that they were not destined to have a baby and got on with their life or who adopted—and then got pregnant. What changes occur in such allegedly infertile people that enable them to become fertile? One thread often linking such stories is that they let go expectation and move to a state akin to resignation, followed by acceptance and eventually reinstatement of a more or less contented way of being. The key point is that the overwhelming stress of wanting and failing is lifted in some way.

Of course there are centuries of mother table-talk on the subject— 'perhaps you are trying too hard, dear' or 'just relax and it will happen'—underlining the simple observation that being uptight or stressed affects our mental and physical status, a natural part of which is our fertility.

Reproductive expert Dr Allen Morgan[9] reinforces the old tales when he says that 'for up to 40 percent of couples, no discernible reason for infertility can be found.' He adds that, 'in this fertile group who don't become pregnant, the effects of stress are most profound.'

What is stress?

More recently, in 2012, Radio National Australia broadcast the results of a survey that suggested 87 percent of people in Australia said that they felt 'stressed'. Although 'stress' is used as a kind of all-purpose word, I suspect that when people use it, they are saying they feel pressured, worried, frustrated, anxious, fretful, troubled . . . enough to have concern that their overall wellbeing is being affected.

Stress consists of three components. Firstly, there is a 'stressor': a demand placed on a person by work, time, financial problems, unemployment, fertility difficulties, pregnancy—almost anything. Then there is the way that demand is perceived, which depends very much on the individual, and, finally, the mind's (and then the body's) response to that stress.

In other words, stress is not definitively quantifiable or scientifically measurable, although psychologists conduct verbal and written tests that they believe show that it is. For example, psych tests tend to suggest that if one gets divorced, moves house, suffers a death in the family—each of which is allocated a certain number of stress points—all in one year, then you will be 'stressed'. Well, yes, one would imagine so.

What is known is that stress is an emotional pressure, which differs from person to person, according to how they respond to the cause of that pressure and the intensity of the pressure itself. Each of us knows what it feels like to be worried or anxious or unhappy. We have all, at some time, had our equanimity trashed by a stressor, whatever that might be. A stressor for one dear friend, for example, was simply being in the presence of seagulls—for another, two years of front-line war.

Stress causes unhealthy tension

Wise ones from yogis to Zen masters through the ages have understood the terrible effects of stress on people. They have long stated that, if stress (emotional burden) is not naturally discharged by having a mature response to a stressor (facing and letting go the issue), pressure dwells in our mind which, in turn and inescapably, has tangible effects on the body. Over time, continuing mental stress is reflected as a physical tension held in the body. If the body is unable to let go that tension, blood flow becomes restricted through non-relaxed muscles, the heart has to beat faster, blood pressure rises and many natural physiological functions, even just elimination, for example, begin to falter until physical or even mental illness sets in—the major clue that we are under siege by a stressor.

In an interview, Nobel prize-winner Dr Elizabeth Blackburn[10] said, '... of course, chronic stress has very profound physiological influences. It is well documented to have clinical effects. There's enough evidence now to show that, for example, it does actually wear down the end of chromosomes. That in turn, wears down the ability of cells to replenish throughout our life which is much of what our body has to do. There is a physical connection between the mind and the body.'

That is the key point, and one that meditation masters have known for centuries. Not only does mental and physical tension age us prematurely, it can cause a whole basketful of other bother along the way. It is now known scientifically that the effects of stress can sneak up on us as headaches, fatigue, intestinal disorders, muscle stiffness and insomnia, as well as anxiety, depression and neuroses.

This has a horrible cyclical effect. The sicker we become, the more we worry. The more we worry, the sicker we become—a physical and mental spiral it is difficult to escape unless some action is taken to combat stress and the consequent mental and physical tension.

Of most importance here, though, is whether there is evidence that such emotional overload has direct implications for a reduction in fertility, difficulties in getting pregnant, and the success or otherwise of IVF programs, all of which, in turn, can cause even further stress.

De-stressing—a solution

Extensive research conducted around the world over the last 20 years by leading universities, hospitals and institutions is now showing compellingly, that de-stressing has a positive effect on 'unexplained' infertility and the success rates of IVF programs.

For example, reflecting much of the research commentary, Dr Allen Morgan says, '20 years ago, the rate of unexplained fertility was between 10 and 20 percent. Today I see up to 40 percent. Women's bodies aren't different, but their stress levels are, and combined with the ticking of the biological clock, I believe it sets the stage for infertility. What we do know now is that, when stress-reduction techniques are employed, something happens in some women that allow them to get pregnant when they couldn't get pregnant before.'

Most of these researchers worldwide are talking of 'relaxation' as the key stress-reduction technique, and it is beginning to be widely recognised medically and scientifically that meditation is the pinnacle of the relaxing techniques. For example, Dr Jamie A Grifo, at the NYU Medical Center in New York City,[11] says that infertility patients are now routinely referred to in-house programs that offer 'guided imagery' (guided meditation or meditative visualization) in an effort to reduce stress.

Deeply encouraging are the studies of Dr Alice Domar of the Harvard Medical School.[12] She has said that, 'reproductive health experts have long wondered about the impact that stress may have on fertility, thus impeding a woman's ability to conceive.' Her research focused on the relationship between stress and different women's health conditions and, as a result, she created innovative programs to help women decrease physical and psychological symptoms of stress.

But there is relatively less formal study on infertility and stress in couples trying to conceive naturally than is being done on seemingly infertile women in IVF programs. The main reason for this is that the seemingly infertile couple doesn't seek medical attention until they have failed to become pregnant for perhaps many months or longer. At that point they may be referred to an IVF program.

Stress and IVF pregnancy

Undergoing IVF, however, can in itself be an immensely stressful time. Professor Dorothy Greenfeld from Yale University says that, 'the stress of actually undergoing infertility treatments can be so great it can stop even the most successful procedure from working.'[13]

Her comment is underlined by an important study presented in 2009 by Dr Alice Domar, showing that when a woman reduces her stress level, she increases the chances that her IVF cycle will be successful.[14] Dr Domar had introduced a mind/body program for infertility,[15] for which the aspiration was to assist couples by training them for 10 weeks in effective relaxation and stress management strategies . . . while attempting to conceive.

Dr Domar found that 52 percent of the women participating in the program became pregnant compared with 20 percent of a control group of participants, a statistically significant difference. She wrote, 'The study shows that here is a strong indication . . . stress levels and IVF outcomes are linked and that intervening with mind/body therapies can help.'

She also found that stress management had an even greater effect on increasing pregnancy rates for women who showed symptoms of depression. Pregnancy rates rose to 67 percent for women with signs of depression who engaged in the stress management program compared with no pregnancies for those who did not.

After two cycles of study, she concluded that those who had 'acquired some real life skills to deal with their stress . . . that's when we saw the significant increase in pregnancy rate.' This study shows that stress management may improve pregnancy rates, minimise the stress of fertility management itself, increase the success rates of IVF procedures and, ultimately, help to alleviate the emotional burden for women who are facing challenges trying to conceive.

Meditation—the ability to release stress

It is not so much the embedding of tension in our body as a result of stress, but rather, the holding on to stress, and our inability to release it, that causes the wide array of fertility challenges listed by Dr Domar.

It is, therefore, mastering the ability to be tension-free that becomes our first base for the mountain climb to true wellbeing.

Using such skilled meditative practices, we can learn to respond positively to the tension-effect of stressors, whatever they are, and develop the ability to just let them go. This natural skill can elevate both our health and our hearts.

At whatever stage of your journey, letting go tension is a major resource in not only aiding pregnancy, but enhancing the motherhood experience throughout. This is the reason that it is the very first meditation practice in Part One.

Meditation—a helping hand with frustration, disappointment and grief

Naturally, trying to become pregnant can lead to frustration, anxiety and stress, in which case stress-relieving practices can be of immense value in enhancing the possibility of falling pregnant. There are some couples, however, who suffer from permanent infertility or lose their child pre-term, experiencing the deepest emotions of sadness, grief and pain.

Meditation is not a magic elixir that eliminates such heartfelt and heart-rending emotions. In fact, really feeling and expressing our sadness is much healthier than bottling it up within and presenting an 'I'm-just-fine-thank-you' face to the world. Such depressing disappointment or loss is life changing, and can ache within for months and years.

I am deeply and personally aware of the pain of loss and the consequent sadness and grief. It may be hard to understand at the time, but know that it does tend to ease as time passes. In fact, there does seem to be a time when we feel the need to move on. As Zen meditation gives us the capacity to delight in our existence, moment by moment, and experience joy and calm, so, when the time is right, individuals and couples experiencing disappointment or loss will slowly realize that they have hearts full of love, care and compassion—hearts still full of giving.

When ready, your job is to honour yourselves—and perhaps a lost one—by passing on the love in so very many possible ways. Giving of our selves with compassionate kindness is actually the ultimate way of lightening our own burdens. Meditation can play a key role in our lives at such times. Practiced with much care of the self, meditation can not only lead you to a place of quietness and peace, but also actually be the light that shows you a way through to . . . passing on the love.

CHAPTER TEN

Meditation and pregnancy: the first trimester

If you have been trying to conceive, hopefully, at some point in your endevor, you will receive the good news from a pregnancy test. From that fertile moment, you have embarked upon a journey . . . an adventure on which you'll not be travelling alone. You have begun creating another being whose life is totally dependent upon yours. You are now the host to a precious embryo, the beginnings of a human, who you will nourish and nurture until she is ready to leave you and begin her own unique life journey.

Over 40 weeks, unseen by you, this child-to-be will draw from your body's wellbeing to cultivate form, function and feelings, all initially shaped by the genes passed to her by both you and your partner. The growth of this embryo into a fetus, from a microscopic single-cell structure to a birth-ready baby, all happens naturally as its development follows the countless commands of the chromosomes and genes drawn from each parent and built into the fertilised egg.

In the following chapters, I will briefly outline the miracle of your baby's growth and development each fortnight in little summary segments headed 'Babywatch'. These will be followed similarly, by a few words in 'Motherwatch', which describes some of the key happenings to your body as the little one grows. Note that my descriptions are quite general. Of course, you are both unique and there may be perfectly normal variations in your development compared with the data in this book. However, all you mums-to-be end up in the same place: holding an angel in your arms

Following these segments there are the Meditation Guidance Panels, which outline the meditation exercises most beneficial to you at each phase of your pregnancy.

Let this wondrous journey begin.

Month 1

When you do find out that you are pregnant, you have been so for at least a month. Those first weeks, and the next six, are the most critical for you and your baby's development. Even though the embryo is only the size of a pinhead embedded in the uterine wall, the placenta and umbilical cord have begun to function, enabling nutrition and oxygen to start being transferred to this tiny life.

In less than four weeks since fertilisation, your embryonic baby will have grown from just one cell to several million cells. The end of the first month is the starting line for an amazing metamorphosis. Whatever you take into your body is being passed to the baby, so you really need to be on full health alert from this exciting moment.

If you have been trying to get pregnant for a while, hopefully you have already introduced your health program and begun the earlier meditation exercises in Part One of this book. But if you haven't, the day you find out that you are having a baby is certainly the day to commence. As this is likely to be early in the second month of your pregnancy, move now to the Meditation Guidance

Panel (page 138) so you can begin the recommended practices.

Month 2

Babywatch

These two weeks are a kind of construction-of-the-foundations stage as the embryo begins to become a fetus – a recognisably human form with a well-organised structure. At a total size of about five millimetres, her head becomes defined but is oversized compared with the body because it becomes the engine room in charge of all the body's developing functions.

The face begins to take shape, organs begin to form and bones, muscles, cartilage and tendons start developing. The arms and legs begin to be defined as buds protruding from the body. At around six weeks, she is about the size of a small bean and her tiny heart is now beating. Embryonic lungs and intestines are beginning to develop.

At around seven weeks, the little one measures about 18 millimetres. Her head is straightening up and, amazingly, most organs are already in place and have begun their lifelong function. The main growth continues to be the brain, where primitive neural pathways are being formed. Weighing in at about 11 or 12 grams at the end of week eight, she is now referred to as a fetus.

Motherwatch

You may notice subtle changes in your second month. One mom-to-be commented that she 'felt her body changing but couldn't see it'. It is possible that a little sickness may be felt in the second month. Your hormones are on the move now (particularly, a rapid increase in progesterone) as your body adjusts to providing a beautifully enriched home for the fetus to live.

All this is an enormous shift in your life, so you may find your emotions fluctuating for a few weeks as you adjust to these hormonal changes. The earlier meditative exercises in letting go tension and breathing in the Meditation Guidance Panel can be very helpful in calming emotional extremes and providing a little extra energy if you feel unusually fatigued and sluggish.

Prenatal screening and testing

Throughout your pregnancy there is a range of diagnostic tests and genetic screening available to you and, as science develops, the tests are increasingly able to tell you more and more about both you and your baby's health. Ask your caregiver about the necessity and purpose of any particular test as many are optional. Some tests, however, such as ultrasound, are considered very important.

Ultrasound

You are likely to have your first ultrasound at about 10 weeks and then every three months. This test is designed to confirm that everything is there and is where it should be. But, as the test is also checking for abnormalities, it can also be a little time of apprehension and anxiety. This is natural, so just use your letting go tension and slow, deep breathing exercises to stay restfully calm. Soon we will see that the baby can actually feel and respond to your emotions, so be happy!

Meditation in Month 2

If you haven't yet started meditating, it is now time. Meditation needs to become a looked-forward-to habit, just like having your first cup of tea of the day.

Have your book, pen and bookmarks with you in your Sanctuary. Keep *Meditation for Motherhood* there so you can bookmark the exercises that you are advised to do in each of the segments as you go along. Leave all of them near your mat when you complete each session and after you have noted the date, length of practice and the exercises completed. This will encourage you to keep going when you don't feel like it, which sometimes you won't.

Very important

At whatever stage you might be in your pregnancy, never do an exercise that makes you uncomfortable in any way or push an activity too far. All the exercises are very gentle and helpful but a few may become a little difficult as you become bigger. For example, very deep breathing is not easy with a big belly. In such instances, I offer alternative, easier exercises that still bring you the full benefit of daily practice. So, throughout your pregnancy, always be patient and gentle with yourself.

Your practice in Weeks 5–6

Total session time: 15 minutes (10 minutes on these exercises, 5 for the breathing practices below)

Exercises 1, 2 and 3 (First Essence—letting go tension)

Notes:

* Do each exercise for two or three days just by itself before progressing. So, you will just do Exercise 1 for three or so days before introducing Exercise 2 . . . and so on. This principle of gentle progress applies throughout your pregnancy. It doesn't matter if you progress a little more quickly or slowly than I suggest.

* These exercises are the beginning of the First Essence, letting go tension. They are done lying down for the first two weeks, just to help you establish a practice pattern.

Add Exercises 8, 9 and 10 (Second Essence—breathing)

Note:

* At this early stage, you add these important breathing exercises after the practices above. You can do them either lying down or sitting.

Your practice in Weeks 7–8

Total session time: 15 minutes divided, as before

Exercises 4, 5, 6 and 7 (Letting go tension)

Notes:

* These exercises are a big step forward. From here on, until later in your pregnancy, try to practice while sitting up. If you practice daily, you may still feel comfortable in the Zen posture until you are birth-ready.

❀ The next big step in this fortnight is beginning to take your practice with you (active meditation) as you go about your daily business. This develops your natural capacity for calmness and lays down skills you can apply later on when you really need them.

Add Exercises 11, 12 and 13 (Beginning right breathing)

Note:

❀ Spend no more than five minutes on these exercises at the moment as they might make you a little dizzy (from taking in a smidge too much oxygen). If this happens, just go back to normal breathing for a while.

❀ As you are going about your day, try and slow your breathing a little whenever you think of it. At the same time, be mindful of breathing into your lower lungs. For example, while sitting at the kitchen table with a cuppa, just pop your hand onto your tummy and practice for a minute or two. Keep taking your skills with you.

Month 3

I have a strange mix of feelings. I want to meet you because I can't see you but feel I already know you.

– BARBARA BACON, MOTHER-TO-BE

Babywatch

During this month, the baby will double in size, growing to between six and seven centimetres and weighing around 20 grams. All her organs are in place, although there is much growing still to come. It is another beautiful month as the brain and nervous system have developed sufficiently to enable her to begin to move, although the movements are just little 'awakening' quivers. By the end of this first trimester, she will be moving freely but you won't detect anything until about five months.

She is now beginning to take on human appearance as the facial features become more distinct. Importantly, the placenta is sufficiently in place to begin one of its tasks—producing hormones. She has most everything now with nerves, muscles and all her organs established in their right place and nutrition flowing directly to her.

She is all set for growing and the vital organs such as the kidneys, intestines and liver begin to function. Her arms are long enough to meet over the chest and legs are able to touch in front of the body. Amazingly, her head is still 50 percent of her body length with a very prominent forehead containing the rapidly expanding brain, which is now directing an increasing storm of growing activity.

The skin is still so fragile it is translucent. Through it, the spine is visible as are the nerves, which begin to travel throughout her body. Movements are becoming graceful but more expansive with kicking and stretching becoming part of her daily repertoire.

Motherwatch

In your third month, the changes in you are not as subtle as they have been. Your uterus will now be the size of a grapefruit and generally, the key changes you'll notice will be an increase in breast and waist size.

Pregnancy sickness usually happens about now, which is not always confined to the mornings. For many women, however, the associated nausea begins to ease before the end of the second trimester and energy levels begin to rise again. Believe it or not, meditation helps to ease nausea.

In this trimester, you may experience an understandably emotional rollercoaster. You may go from feeling extremely elated to apprehensive, all involved with your confidence about becoming a mother. This is quite common in the first trimester and tends to diminish in the second but may reoccur in the third as the time gets closer. Your meditation can really, really help you at this time.

Keep on with your physical exercises. Maintaining fitness will strengthen you to help you carry the impending extra weight without too much strain. Exercise is now an important part of your daily routine and also a partial shield against emotional disturbance. Being fit now is also a wonderful base from which to work in getting back to 'match-ready status' after the birth.

Meditation in Month 3

Your practice in Weeks 9–10

Total session time: 15 minutes

For a good month or more now, you have been developing two of the most important practices in meditation: letting go tension and slow, deep (*hara*) breathing, which will be coming increasingly natural to you. You are ready to move on.

Exercise 14 (Practicing the first two Essences together)

Notes:

❄ In this exercise, we combine the first two Essences to strengthen the base for adding the Third Essence (quieting the mind) and later, meditating.

❄ So, for the next two weeks, I just want you to practice this exercise.

Important: Having mastered this practice to a reasonable level, it then becomes your natural prelude to **all** further exercises and meditation. So, assume 'Exercise 14' is written at the beginning of every exercise and meditation you practice from here on until it becomes second nature to you.

Your practice in Weeks 11–12

Total session time: increase to 20 minutes

Continue Exercise 14 (Practicing the first two Essences together)

Add Exercise 15 (Whole-body breathing)

Notes:

❀ In Week 11, add on this deeper exercise and give full attention to it for about the last five minutes before completing so that, after a week, you are able to do whole-body breathing competently. You will find this a wonderfully refreshing practice and invaluable for later on.

❀ Before completing the session, just return to gentle *hara* breathing for a minute or two.

❀ From the second trimester onwards, you need only incorporate this exercise into your practice about once a week.

Add Exercises 16 and 17 (Dynamic breathing and breathing walks)

Notes:

- ❋ Add these when you are ready, but about this time is ideal. Start very gently and gradually build your capacity. You can practice dynamic breathing more strenuously when exercising or walking, or more gently within any meditation.

- ❋ Hopefully, walking is now part of your exercise regimen. By adding Exercise 16, you can begin using your walks as meditation practice.

- ❋ Practice dynamic breathing until it becomes natural as it is most valuable during labor.

Filomena's story

Hardship during pregnancy

After five years of trying to conceive, many operations later and two cycles of IVF, my husband and I were finally having a baby. Having gone through IVF, we had seen our little one twice before the normal 12-week scan.

We were so happy and, at the 12-week scan, everything seemed to be going fine until we were given the news that our baby had a birth defect. It was a *cystic hygroma*, a growth that often occurs in the head and neck area. Our world came crashing down and a sense of despair and fear overwhelmed me. I could not imagine having to terminate the pregnancy.

My saving grace was meditation, which I had been practicing daily for about four weeks at that stage and was still attending sessions at the Meditation Sanctuary in Rozelle with Brahm. My daily meditation gave me the calmness and strength to face the road ahead.

It almost felt as though I was watching someone else's violent storm out in the ocean. Even though the storm around me was my own and so violent, it never came close enough to harm me and I felt an overwhelming sense of peace and calmness. I also decided to visualize daily that my baby was perfectly healthy and normal. My daily meditation practice over the next five weeks carried me through this difficult stage.

At 17 weeks, we at last received the results from the amniocentesis that our little angel was perfectly normal and thriving with no signs of a *cystic hygroma* or any other birth defect. I'm now 28 weeks along and continuing this wonderful journey of serenity.

I hope my story serves as some inspiration to other moms around the world who may be facing similar hardships during their pregnancy. I was so appreciative of my teacher's help, support, and words of wisdom along with the great stories of encouragement in every meditation class.

Beautiful baby Claudio was born at full term and greeted the world safely and well.

CHAPTER ELEVEN

Meditation and pregnancy: the second trimester

The special feature of this trimester is the great sense of bonding that develops between you and your baby because you become aware of her moving. As her senses develop, you begin to share emotions and sensations as she becomes responsive to sound vibrations and movements transmitted through the amniotic fluid.

In this, the second trimester, as your baby bump begins to appear, the little one develops all the features of a newborn with the size of her body beginning to play catch-up with the head, now only a third of her body length. The good news for you is that your pregnancy sickness will either diminish or completely disappear.

Month 4

Babywatch

Your little angel is awakening. The key development continues to be in her brain, with thousands of neurons appearing every minute and continuing to link with each other. The brain is now sending out constant electrical and chemical signals. At birth, she will have the most complex computer in the world in her head, with around 100 billion neurons and a million billion connections between them— the home for all her senses and emotions.

She now begins resting occasionally for a few seconds before moving again, the beginning of sleep. By the end of this month, her body and limbs will start to become sensitive to touch and her movements become increasingly refined. Around Week 14, her face shows an increasing repertoire of expressions such as frowning, squinting and grimacing.

The placenta has become an exquisitely efficient filter that allows small particles of nutrients, proteins and sugar fats to pass to your baby but blocks out larger, harmful particles such as bacteria. Your own health is increasingly important for her health.

At the end of Week 14, she is about the length of your palm and weighs 65 grams.

The story of wonderment continues. The primitive air sacs in the lungs expand and her sense of sight has developed to a point where she would move to avoid bright light. Although there is not much on the menu yet, her little taste buds have begun developing too. These two weeks are the beginning of a rapid growing period lasting several weeks, during which she will double her weight and length.

Motherwatch

You are probably feeling better now with less nausea and your moods are becoming more balanced again. This can be a time of experiencing a lovely sense of wellbeing as your energy returns. It is in the latter part of this month that you may begin to feel her movements. They are actually vigorous from her point of view but tiny in relation to your body. Some women say that the early movements are like having bubbles in the tummy or a tiny worm wriggling around.

She is increasingly sensitive to what you are doing as her senses develop. For example, if you do vigorous exercise, so does she. The baby's movements will increase and her heart rate will rise to up to 220 beats a minute, only settling back to her standard 160 when you stop. Conversely, as I mentioned earlier, she may also meditate when you do.

So, from this month on, with her senses developing, there is a direct correlation between your state of being and that of your baby's. In other words, your emotional state (which can affect heart rate, hormonal output, blood pressure and so on) is also transmitted to the baby.

You are now eating for two. So listen to your body as it tells you to let go junk food and take your fill of balanced, nutritious meals. Refer to expert advice for the right amounts of protein, iron, vitamins, minerals and particularly calcium (for her bones and teeth) you now need.

Meditation in Month 4

Given that your emotional state now affects the baby, your meditation becomes increasingly important. Although you will introduce some new exercises this month and begin the Third Essence, quieting the mind, it is imperative to continue the first two—letting go tension and slow *hara* breathing. These have the greatest positive effect throughout your pregnancy and are a 'meditative must' for delivery.

Your practice in Weeks 13–14

Total session time: Up to 25 minutes now please, including about 5 minutes for beginning the Third Essence (below)

Continue Exercises 14 and 15 (Practicing the first two Essences and whole-body breathing)

Important: physical exercise and meditation

I recommend that you now separate your physical exercises and meditation practice by half an hour because it is time to introduce some extra lung-strengthening and breath-control work. Some of these new breathing exercises can be quite vigorous in your early stages, so incorporating them in your actual exercise programme is the best time for them. I am suggesting separating exercise and meditation because, quite simply, it is difficult to settle into meditation immediately after physical activity or to begin strenuous work immediately following the calmness of meditation.

Add Exercises 18–21 (Lung cleansing and strengthening)

Notes:

* Follow the instructions carefully about progressing these exercises slowly so you don't overdo them.

* Remember, quiet body and quiet breathing (Essences one and two) are the base practices with which you now commence all exercises and meditations.

Your practice in Weeks 15–16

Total session time: 30 minutes for the Three Essences

Exercise 22 (Learning to focus thoughts using a mantra)

Notes:

❀ This practice alone is very calming because it centres your focus on just one point. For this whole week, allocate 10 minutes to the first two Essences before introducing the mantra. The secret to successfully focusing on a mantra is being aware when your mind wanders and gently bring it back to 'just this'.

❀ In situations of anxiety or stress, you can practice active meditation by just saying your mantra, either in your mind (wherever you are) or even aloud. You will find yourself calming because you can't get too lost in thought if you are busy focusing on a soothing mantra. Remember this for later on in the whole birthing activity.

❀ Refer back to the list of lovely mantras in Part One, on page 82.

Exercise 23 (Beginning meditation proper—letting go techniques)

Notes:

❀ Be very patient and follow the guidelines. This exercise may take some time to master but even moments of stillness in the early stages are to be celebrated.

❀ Practice your walking meditation and dynamic breathing several times a week if you can.

Month 5

The angel is growing and now beginning what I call her 'enter-tainment' phase. In this month, she is increasingly human in appearance (exquisitely so) and really becoming creative in her activities. Ultrasounds have shown little ones holding onto the umbilical cord and even pulling their feet up to put their toes in their mouth.

You may begin to find your exercises require greater effort. Your pregnancy is now top priority in your life and some women choose to begin slowing down a little. Naturally, everyone's experience will differ and whatever you feel is right for you, is right for you.

Babywatch

Her senses are developing so she is becoming sensitive to the taste of the amniotic fluid, which has its own unique aromatic composition as a result of the foods eaten by you. As her smell receptors and tastebuds are linked to the brain, the information she is getting from her liquid environment is beginning to build her memory bank of tastes and smells. Prenatal researchers such as Benoist Schaal, say that the baby's later preference for certain foods is actually formed at this time.

Of great interest is her beginning to detect your voice resonating as vibration through her home bubble, although it is more felt through the sense of touch rather than hearing, which doesn't fully develop until much closer to birth. (See segment on page 164 at the end of Motherwatch in Month 8 on how a fetus in the womb learns through her hearing sense before birth and, accordingly, whether mother-stress affects the baby.) Around the last week of this month, she is about the size of a banana—16 centimetres or so. This seems a rather sudden leap except that, from Week 20, she is now measured from head to toes because her legs can stretch out quite fully.

Motherwatch

You might notice an increase in your appetite, which is normal as long as you are maintaining a good balance in your nutrition. Your body now needs more iron to keep up with your expanding blood volume, so make sure that your diet is catering for this. You might also experience a little pain in your lower tummy. This is likely to be caused by ligaments stretching to accommodate the weight of an increasingly heavy uterus.

Week 20 . . . you are halfway there!

I mentioned that baby can now detect sounds as vibrations and experts believe that you can begin bonding with the baby by talking to her. I also suggest you make soft, warm sounds such as repeating *OM* or *AUM* as a gentle mantra (see your new meditation practices at the end of this section), which produce rhythmic vibrations in the fluid surrounding her. Calmness is so important now because, as I discuss later, she is actually able to identify whether your mood is happy or sad and can be affected accordingly.

Meditation in Month 5

Your practice in Weeks 17–18

Total session time: 30 minutes

Exercises 24 and 25 (A mantra for your baby)

Stay with this practice for two weeks and also introduce some additional work on mindfulness soon.

Notes:

❋ Turning your mind mantra into a vocalised mantra (in other words, saying it out loud) has two purposes:

  – firstly, you can use it to quieten your mind just as you did with the mind mantra

  – secondly, whenever you want to communicate with the baby, you can hum or repeat your mantra out loud to her, soothing her by the vibration of your now-familiar voice. Encourage your partner to speak or sing to the little one who, in the womb, will learn this second familiar source of sound.

A little author story

I practiced this second exercise on my treasured first-born son, from the day he came home. I would hold his ear against my chest and just hum softly or chant AUM. He would soon fall asleep. He grew up to be a beautiful singer, composer and musician. That may, of course, be just a coincidence or . . . maybe not.

Add Exercises 31 and 32 (Awakening the senses—the wonderment of mindfulness)

Note:

❋ These practices are in addition to your sitting meditation. You can commence them anytime this month.

Your practice in Weeks 19–20

In this fortnight, simply continue practicing the Three Essences as well as using the mantra to quieten your mind. But when you feel ready, you can begin to introduce another technique below.

Continue your practice of mindfulness, which you can begin to take with you at any time. Mindfulness is the masterly and wonderful way to bring yourself to 'just now' and lift you away from anxiety or apprehension.

Exercises 26 and 27 (Breathing—used as a technique to focus the mind)

Note:

❀ From now, you can choose any technique to quieten your mind before then letting it go so you can dwell in silence. When you find one that works for you, settle on it rather than exploring them all.

Month 6

Babywatch

By the end of this month she really resembles a little human, but there is much development still to go before she is birth-ready, so the growth spurt continues. The early bubbles and flutters of movement have now become the fully fledged kicks and punches of a mini martial artist. Her senses continue to develop. For example, sound passing through the amniotic fluid will actually make the little eardrums vibrate. She can hear.

Sometime during this month, she will open her eyes. The pigment of her irises hasn't been created yet but, as with most babies, they are most likely to be blue when she is born. They may stay blue or, if she is to have another color, the change will occur in the months after birth. Her senses will be set at 'all systems go' at birth, except for her eyesight, which will continue maturing for at least another six weeks.

The baby's skeleton is still growing and, incredibly, she will have 300 bones at full term so her little body is flexible enough to be born. Once in the world, some bones begin to fuse and, as an adult, she will have only 206.

Her lungs are preparing for breathing and cells in them are producing a substance that will help the alveoli (little air sacs) to inflate when she takes that miraculous first breath. By month's end, she'll be about 30 centimetres at full stretch (not too many vegies this big to compare her with—try a large carrot or ear of corn).

Motherwatch

You are not overly big just yet, but noticeably 'with child'. There will be significant changes in you over the next couple of months, but you are probably feeling quite comfortable.

You can still do physical work and exercise but it is time to begin gradually easing the pace of both. You can keep walking as a wonderful exercise until the day she is born, although jogging five laps of the oval is definitely out.

Because of pregnancy hormones, you may notice that your skin is more beautiful. Your hair may seem to be more lustrous and actually thicker. It's not as a result of growing more—it's just that you are losing less. Your fingernails may also grow more quickly. All these, and indeed any little negative changes such as excess body hair, will all return to normal after the birth. You can still enjoy intercourse using appropriately gentle positions virtually until birth-time.

Your tummy is expanding to make room for the baby so you may get tissue striations, known as stretch marks. Your nipples and areolas (the circular area around your nipples) will also be getting darker and larger. There are also pronounced bumps on the areolas. These are little glands that produce oils that fight bacteria and lubricate the skin.

You may experience fluid retention, which will most likely disappear within days of her arrival. Contrary to expectation, drinking more water helps prevent fluid retention.

Meditation in Month 6

Your practice in Weeks 21–22

Total session time: up to 40 minutes

Exercises 28 and 29 (Opening eyes meditation—deepening focus)

Notes:

❀ I am suggesting longer times for your formal practice now. I know that your comfort factor will begin to be an issue so you may wish to do two half-sessions rather than one longer one.

❀ This is the beginning of meditation with open eyes. It really is a significant practice in mastering your focus and being able to calm yourself with your eyes open. It can be an invaluable practice for birthing time.

Add Exercises 33 and 34 (Mind settling—wherever you are)

Notes:

❀ The important aspect of your practice now is not confining it to your sanctuary but, increasingly, taking it with you.

- This fortnight, the practice is to begin increasing awareness of your thinking as you go about your business. As you know, when you master that, you're more settled emotionally.

Your practice in Weeks 23–24

Total session time: 40 minutes

Exercise 30 (Full meditation with open eyes—letting go the technique)

Notes:
- This is one of the amazing skills in meditation. I have brought it in now so you have much time to work with it.
- If you prefer your daily practice with closed eyes, that is just fine. But practice a full open-eyes meditation about once a week or so, because much of your time in the birthing room will be with your eyes open.

Exercises 35 and 36 (Leading a more meditative life)

Note:
- When you have time, study these gentle, natural practices and gradually introduce them at your own pace over the remaining weeks. You will find them invaluable.

Filomena's story

Meditation and calmness after a fall

Twenty weeks pregnant exactly and all was going well until I fell.
I missed a step on my staircase, lost my balance and went flying. As I was trying not to fall flat on my belly, I managed to pull my left leg forward when I reached the floor of the dining room. My knee and lower back took the full impact of the fall.

I felt my belly tense up so tight I thought I was going to go into labor. My knee and back were hurting. I managed to get myself to my couch and all I could think of was to lie perfectly still and focus on my breathing and to redirect my breathing to my belly, knee and lower back. I was using one of the practices I learned at the Meditation Sanctuary. My body began to relax and I could feel the tension in my belly completely subside and no longer felt the pain in my knee and lower back.

After lying on the couch doing 'right' breathing for a good hour or more, I could feel the baby happily moving around. I was advised to go to the emergency unit to be sure no harm had come to my baby and to get myself checked too. It turned out all was fine with the little one and my placenta was unharmed—no amniotic leakage either. As for me, I had no bruising or swelling in my knee and no harm was done to my back. For the first time ever, I didn't need to take any painkillers. The next day I was at my weekly meditation class!

As I have, I think you can give yourself the greatest and most wonderful gift that will help you through, not only your pregnancy but, every aspect of your life by practicing Zen meditation.

CHAPTER TWELVE

Meditation and pregnancy: the third trimester

You have turned the corner into the third and last trimester and every passing day she spends nestled in your womb is adding to her strength and maturity. She is readying herself for a grand entrance into the world. The emphasiz in this trimester is to ensure that she grows to full term. This offers her the best possible opportunity for complete health and wellbeing. Your calmness and caring for you both becomes your priority in life.

Month 7

Babywatch

Your little one has been turning somersaults (there's not a lot else for her to do) but these begin to slow down and eventually stop because she is now filling most of the space available in her liquid home. She is getting ready to turn upside down to be in position for the birth – you are very likely to feel this magical moment when it happens.

Her little lungs continue to develop and she actually practices 'breathing' by inhaling and exhaling amniotic fluid. The nervous system is nearing completion and she makes distinct facial expressions ranging from complete tranquillity to frowning. She will exercise her arms and legs rhythmically as if lifting weights— all strengthening her muscles.

The network of nerves in her ears continues to develop and she can hear the muffled sounds of your conversations increasingly clearly.

My 'development reports' become briefer from now on, as your precious one is basically busy just putting on weight and adding the finishing touches. Her brain is extremely active and still growing more tissue and adding millions more neurons. She is sleeping regularly but, when awake, frequently opens and closes her eyes and probably detects different intensities of light that filter into your womb.

At the end of this month, she will measure about 32 centimetres from head to heels and weigh up to one kilogram. Given that the average baby weight is a little over three kilograms at birth, you can see that her main activity in this last trimester is developing baby fat.

Motherwatch

Your lovely mother-body is beginning to prepare for birth. Baby knows exactly what she is doing and has herself well organised. For the next couple of months, just allow everything to proceed quietly and naturally, doing what you can easily. Rest and meditate more to ensure growing calmness and the refinement of your focus for the big event.

Continue a balanced fitness program including mother-to-be yoga, walking and swimming if possible. Maintaining fitness, muscle tone and general body strength is really important because you are under strain and may be getting more tired now as so much energy and nutrition is being drawn from you by the junior athlete.

There are many ways to overcome or alleviate late pregnancy discomforts. Again, your careperson is the best one with whom to chat. Common sense will get you most of the way, however, and a gentle program of self-care is top of your list for the rest of the journey.

The respected French midwife Francine Dauphin[16] recommends a visit to the birthing place about this time, to familiarise yourself with the environment and to meet the people who are likely to be helping at delivery. She emphasizes good birth preparation, although she says there is 'no ticket to a perfect delivery' but a 'good preparation . . . is when a woman feels good!'

She also suggests spending time with a qualified and caring midwife (or appropriate healthcare-giver) who can help you with advice and knowledge on the important things so there are no sudden surprises. The more you know about your body and the birthing process, the more at peace you will be.

There is no ultimate way of preparing. I feel the ultimate knowledge is deep within. The baby knows what to do and when to do it and she is really inviting you to participate, cooperate and assist. Your task in preparing is to accept her invitation with joy and peacefulness.

Meditation in Month 7

Your practice in Weeks 25–28

Total session time: 45–60 minutes

From now on, I'll just make brief comment on the overall month's practice because you know all the core meditative exercises of body, breathing and mind and are hopefully being as mindful as possible. It is time to use your 'dwelling' ability to spend the next two or three months putting your meditation to work in helping you prepare for labor and delivery.

Exercises 37–40 (Using visualization)

Note:

- ✸ These are several preparatory exercises to do before you move to visualizing the birth. Really give time to these exercises. It will make the key visualization much more effective in easing your birthing apprehension when you actually begin practicing it soon.

Month 8

Babywatch

The final touches on the internal organs continue as well as the maturing of her muscles and lungs. The brain is still getting bigger and, to accommodate it, so is her head. Her skeleton is hardening so her uptake of calcium from your body is magnifying. It is a time now of really rapid growth and filling out.

Although her eyesight is far from 20/20 at birth, she will be able to see objects about 10 or 15 centimetres away and so, importantly, will be able to see your face. She already knows you intimately through her developed sense of taste and hearing, which will be an immediate comfort from her first breath.

Because she is occupying most of the uterus, her movements are more restricted but she will be very active, as you will notice because her kicks can be so strong they may interrupt your sleep. This is a good sign that she is fit, healthy and rearing to go.

After her long journey so far, in the next seven or so weeks she will put on about half her birth weight. About now, she will tip the scales at around 1.5 kilos and be approximately 38 centimetres long.

Motherwatch

Given the baby's additional demands, especially for calcium, you will need to give special attention to your own nutrition, making sure you get plenty of calcium, iron, protein, vitamin C and folic acid.

As you grow outwards, you will be less comfortable as she pushes ever upwards into your own tummy area. Again, most symptoms are alleviated with common-sense responses, from a high-fibre diet to regular exercise and drinking lots of water.

At this time, if you rise too quickly from a lying position, you may get a little dizzy, so now is the time for gentle, graceful movements (which will be happening more anyway if you have been calming daily with your meditation).

You may find the mood swings that you experienced early in your pregnancy are tending to wander back again. This can be caused by a combination of reasons, from tiredness, ongoing hormonal changes and moments of apprehension over the journey in front of you still to be faced. This is all normal, but if you are worried or 'getting the blues' about anything at all, share the issue with your partner and professionals. Again, just sitting and quieting yourself daily with meditation can be of enormous benefit.

One feature of being this far along is the possibility of having random little contractions (tightenings of the uterus). They are called Braxton Hicks contractions and can happen at just about any time in the second half of the pregnancy. They are painless and irregular and may last up to about 30 seconds.

If they begin to happen frequently, even if painless, or you have several in an hour, immediately contact your doctor as a precaution. They can be the symptoms of pre-term labor along with menstrual-like cramping, pressure in the pelvic area and lower back pain.

There are only a few weeks to go. Approach difficulties with deliberate, thoughtful slowness and gently experiment with easier ways to do things. You have time, because life is now about you and your baby.

Hearing awareness and baby's response to mother-stress

I have given special emphasiz to this segment because it underlines the evidence of the importance of your stress management on the short- and long-term wellbeing of your baby.

A key question that has fascinated scientists worldwide is: just how much can a fetus hear and what effect does a variety of sounds have on the little one? For example, do soothing sounds quieten the baby and, conversely, do sharp, argumentative sounds (and consequent physiological changes in the mother such as higher blood pressure and faster heartbeat) have an effect on the baby's wellbeing? In other words, do babies respond to either calmness or stressfulness in mothers?

Not all these vital questions have been answered yet, but professional studies continue to be undertaken around the world. Ultimately, scientists are interested in how prenatal experience may help an infant get a 'head start' on developing a language and becoming a competent human being.

I take this a little further by postulating that a woman who is settled and calm throughout pregnancy and birth produces a calmer, more settled child, which is more likely to have positive implications for the rest of her life.

At around the end of the eighth month, the baby's hearing is quite well developed. She reacts to mother-sounds which, in her world, are essentially your heartbeat and digestive sounds.

Hearing specialist and developmental psychobiologist Carolyn Granier-Deferre[17] says that the baby 'will also hear its mother's voice via the tissues and bones. The fetus can probably hear low-pitched sounds because they go straight through the body. On the other hand, very high-pitched sounds get amplified. The mother's womb is like an echo chamber. For instance, if someone is having a conversation (a normal conversation is around 60 decibels) . . . the fetus gets 30 decibels. Now 20 to 30 decibels is equivalent to a whisper . . . just audible to it.' And Granier-Deferre says further that the baby at this stage reacts (with facial expressions) particularly to the mother's voice 'which she is gradually learning to recognise.'

Love that Beethoven!

Graniere-Deferre also showed that babies recognise and respond to music played to them in the womb.[18] She played a descending piano melody to fetuses at Weeks 35, 36 and 37. When the same music was played to them a month after birth, their heart rates calmed by 12 beats per minute compared with a control group whose hearts slowed by only six beats per minute. So, if your baby calls out, 'Love that Beethoven!' then you know you have something very special brewing in there.

French researchers are pioneering the field of prenatal hearing and baby's linguistic awareness in the weeks before, and just after, birth. Aurelie Ribeiro of the University of Paris[19] conducted an experiment aimed at testing whether a fetus can differentiate between words, noise and music. She consistently played to a fetus his Icelandic mother's words and sounds with the same melody and tempo until, whenever it was played, the baby's heart rate would slow because he was familiar with his mother's voice and language. He was being lulled by a calm, familiar sound.

Then an unfamiliar sharper sound such as running water was added. Ribeiro found that 'when we introduced the sound, the heart rate increased. This means the fetus felt the change. So it can differentiate between a short syllabic phrase and a short noisy phrase.'

The research means quite simply that the fetus can not only hear its mother's voice while in the womb but also differentiate between sounds from melodic to sharp, to a point where its heart rate is affected.

Professor Anthony DeCasper of the University of North Carolina[20] studies memory and learning development by assessing the impact of voices the baby has learned in the uterus. He does this immediately after their birth. He developed experiments that involved babies sucking on a mock nipple that was connected to a computer which, in turn, could register the speed the baby sucked. The baby was fitted with earphones for the experiment. When the baby sucked slowly, one sound was played through the earphones and vice versa. DeCasper's findings are astonishing. He proved that newborn babies:

* took just five minutes to learn which sounds they preferred to hear
* identified their mother immediately by sucking faster on hearing her voice and slower if they heard the voice of another woman
* would suck faster in order to hear their mother.

Professor DeCaspar concluded that, to know her mother's voice, the young one must have learned to differentiate it in the womb. By using the nipple technique, he also discovered that a newborn remembered:

* a speech pattern that a mother had been asked to repeat over and over before the baby was born and then

recorded and played to them through their headphones (indicated by a fast sucking, positive response)

❧ those identical speech patterns or language signals if repeated by another person.

Studies in France subsequently proved that babies did indeed know the difference between, say, French and Russian and even showed preference for the language they 'liked better' which, if they were French, was French and vice versa. So babies are born already able to identify both the voice and the national language of their mother.

Your baby understands and responds to your moods

So what practical value might all this uplifting research offer the expectant woman?

For me, the most amazing revelation from the research supports the practice of meditation during pregnancy. This follows from the evidence that the newborn is able to tell whether you speak in a happy or sad way. She actually understands and responds to your moods as soon as she is born, which means that, in the womb, she has already developed awareness of your emotions and mood changes.

Professor DeCaspar was able to show this by exposing babies to different emotions in different languages. He said, 'if you . . . say some words in French as if you are happy and then if you say exactly the same words as if you are sad . . . French babies (for example) can tell the difference between those two emotions. But if you ask a German baby, "Can you tell the difference between the moods of the French speaker?" the answer is "no". They would not be able to do that without that (womb) experience of their mother's language.'

So know that by the end of the eighth month, your bonding with your baby has already begun. You are in the process of becoming a family in a most real sense, before she is born.

I feel strongly that if every new parent-to-be was aware of just how sensitive their little one is to language and emotion, the air would be full of love, softness and gentle words just about the whole time.

Meditation in Month 8

Your practice in Weeks 29–32

Total session time: 45–60 minutes

Exercises 41 and 42 (Visualizing the main journey)

Notes:

❀ At this stage, it is probably a good idea to jump forward for 10 minutes and read over the labor and delivery segments so that you can refine your practice to align with your likely needs then. In those segments, I do make suggestions on which meditations are likely to be of most value to you, but the decisions are yours to make. Just ensure that your skills in letting go tension, right breathing and focusing are being sharpened on a daily basis.

❀ If you read through the baby-awareness segment on pages 164 and 169, you will understand that it is probably a good idea to spend a lot of time now humming, saying your mantra aloud or speaking and singing very softly and melodically to her.

Exercise 43 (Smiling meditation)

No comments necessary.

Month 9

Babywatch

She is just about ready. She now looks like a little human ready to hit the ground running as her skeleton continues to harden. Her fat is layering under beautifully smooth skin so she can regulate her body temperature after birth. The complex nervous system and lungs are undergoing the finishing touches for birth readiness. With five or so weeks to go, she is almost 45 centimetres long and probably around 2.5 kilos.

By the end of Week 38, she is considered full-term (which is really anywhere between 37 and 40 weeks) and is packing her bags. Just for fun, though, she will keep you guessing at her arrival time and will come along just when she's ready. She is almost certainly in the head-down position ready for birth.

Motherwatch

Just as she is about ready, so are you. You feel and act heavily pregnant. Your normally graceful, balletic walk is no more and doing almost anything is increasingly less comfortable. This really is the time for full attention to you. Experiment to find the most comfortable ways to do things. Rest as much as you are able but still get some exercise—quiet walking, slow water aerobics and the gentlest yoga are still all fine. Maintain your soothing communication with your little one and keep going with your daily meditation.

You have up to a month to go, so now is the time to finalise arrangements for going to the birthing place and who you want with you, if anyone other than your partner.

Month 10

Babywatch

Nothing really new happens from now except that she continues to grow until reaching her birth weight (boys are likely to be a little heavier than girls).

She is still fattening up and at birth (as an average) is likely to weigh about 3.5 kilos and be approximately 50 centimetres at full stretch.

Motherwatch

At some time this month, probably more towards the end, you are likely to go into labor, although there is no way to accurately predict when this will be. You may experience a show, your waters may break or contractions may become regular. When the contractions get to be about a minute long and are occurring about every five minutes for an hour, it is time to contact the birthplace and tell your chauffeur to pack the car. It is then time to head off.

If you go beyond time, some practitioners will let you wait for nature to take its course if they determine that all is well with you both. Somewhere before 42 weeks, however, you are likely to be induced when the risk of not giving birth is greater than being induced.

Whatever way it happens for you, at this time I want you happy, peaceful and able to let go any twinges of apprehension virtually at will now, because it won't be long before the pregnancy (and delivery) will be relegated to memory as you gaze upon the loveliest little face you've ever seen.

Meditation in Months 9 and 10

Total session time: 60 minutes or as much as you can. Vary session times as you wish.

Note:

❀ The key from herein until delivery is deep calmness. Concentrate your practice on letting go tension at will, the breathing variations and on the focusing exercises. With your meditation and visualization skills, you can be confident that you have the best tools available to humankind to achieve this. Keep using and enjoying them.

CHAPTER THIRTEEN

Meditation and preparation for the birth

There are so many things to plan in preparing to become a bigger family. There are a number of issues that may be resolved and certainly some activities that can be made less burdensome by applying your meditation skills. Ahead of time, you may actually want to write in your meditation diary the matters you need to consider, the tasks to be done and allocate them to a particular month.

In planning ahead, you will immediately lift one of the major stress burdens from your shoulders—the last-minute rush or the 'oh-my-god-I-forgot-to' problems.

Familiarisation

A real comfort for you and your partner is familiarising yourselves with everything, from the best route to the hospital to the layout of the birthing room itself. Try a full dry-run from home to the birthing place. Most hospitals and birthing facilities have guided tours, so book in for one and ask all the questions you wish about the facilities available.

Meditation practice for the trip to the birthplace

During a dry-run trip, practice being calm by letting go tension and breathing as slowly and as deeply as you comfortably can. Let you movements be gentle and graceful, all of which add to calmness. You are creating a mental blueprint for the main event.

What to take with you

Prepare a list within your meditation diary of everything you think you'll need to take with you because you may be confined for several days. Run a second column for your partner because he could be with you for many hours without much of a break. Above all, list your soothing meditation items such as:

* your favourite object for open-eyes meditation
* a beautiful stone for holding, touching and squeezing to bring you back to 'just this' (it also saves breaking the bones in your partner's hands!)
* calming music and sounds such as the sea, humming, chanting, shakuhachi flute, chimes and bells
* a music player with headset to drown out distractions
* a bottle of a soothing aroma (such as pachouli) and incense if you wish (check if this is permitted).

Meditation and communication

Remind your partner that you will be practicing meditation for much of the time, from travelling to the birthplace through to the end of delivery and beyond. Perhaps suggest that he read this book as well so that he understands the value of, and reasons for, your meditation work.

Most importantly, tell hospital staff (and any other involved people) that you will be meditating during the labor and birth, particularly in the later stages, and explain your preference for chatter and noise being kept to a minimum. Ask your partner ahead of time to play your guardian angel, quieting others if they are too loud. Just like a meditation sanctuary, the quieter the environment, the calmer the people.

Who should be with you at the birth

Giving birth is a most intimate and intensely personal experience and many just want to share it with their partner. Others may want a family member or professional assistant with them. If you have a specialist assistant, make sure your partner is welcomed to participate in personal and special ways (soothing, hugging, kissing, fetching—you've got the idea).

Visitors

I suggest you tell family and others of your visiting wishes beforehand. Being visited while in labor robs you of your precious meditation time. In some countries, however, the mother-people are the key ones who do everything, from encouraging to delivering. But always remember that you are totally in charge of your needs at this time.

Birth plan and issues to consider

Many commentators across the medical spectrum suggest you create a 'birth plan'—writing down your thoughts of how you would like the birth to progress. It is an excellent way to clarify what you ideally want and why, and helps you to focus your mind on your intentions.

There are various issues that you and you partner may need to consider, whether written into a birth plan or not. I will discuss some of the various options you may choose to think over, but know that any decisions are yours and yours alone, drawn from your inner wisdom.

Natural or assisted birth

. . . deliveries, these days . . . are way too technical. Technology is everywhere... and the women, in France, are so conditioned, they think that without technology they can't do it . . . especially without an epidural. So, I say, it is all too much. After thousands of years of deliveries, you wonder how so many children have been born. We should give it some thought and some thinking is being done. My struggle is not for an ideology of delivery, not to say 'this is the right way', but to allow choice.

– FRANCINE DAUPHIN, FRENCH ACTIVIST AND MIDWIFE

To have a natural or assisted birth is really the key question in your planning. Although some labors and deliveries don't go to plan and require medical intervention, the significant majority do, or could, go naturally as intended. On the basis that yours then has a greater chance of progressing normally than not, it is wise to plan what kind of birth you prefer so that when the time comes, as best possible, delivery occurs as you wished it.

There are mountains of opinion on the value or otherwise of natural birth and, similarly, on taking pain-relieving drugs, having an epidural, having a planned induction or a planned cesarean section. Of course, any of the above variations may occur either because of known conditions or unexpected complications.

I make brief comment on them because, firstly, the noticeably positive effects of your meditation (if you have been practicing daily) may well have given you an inner confidence to make such important decisions with a clear, focused mind.

Secondly, if you choose to have a natural birth, you know early on to continue honing your meditative skills because they become powerful weapons to help you remain calm, deeply focused and better able to manage pain. For a practiced person, meditation can potentially become a replacement for taking drugs or having an epidural or, as a minimum, be a potent support system for you.

Natural birth

Fear of childbirth has become a modern day epidemic amongst pregnant women. Childbirth is a natural, normal, life-changing event and, while sometimes intervention may be required in order for a safe outcome for you and/or your baby, birth is not automatically a medical event the moment you fall pregnant.

– Kelly Wider [21]

This is a birthing attitude that seems to have arisen with advances in technology. But we tend to forget that, up until about a century ago, all births were virtually natural. As one mother said to me, 'I needed to tell people to stop pandering to me because I am just pregnant, not sick.'

Kelly Wider says further that 'many of us have found . . . a lack of support, education and encouragement to help women achieve the natural birth they hope for. Not only that, labor pain . . . is being seen by some as "unnecessary" or "bad" pain—when it is, in fact, a very useful pain.' Indeed, in the western world there tends to be an attitude that no-one needs to suffer in childbirth or have their planned lives disrupted by not knowing exactly when the baby is due.

Wider found, however, that an increasing number of women are choosing to have a natural birth. In the simplest of evidence for this, over the last decade of my teaching, I have observed more and more pregnant women attending the Meditation Sanctuary to make calming and focusing skills a centrepiece of their journey through pregnancy, labor and birth. Ten years ago, about two pregnant women a year learned meditation at our Sanctuary but that number has grown to one or two in most classes.

Some benefits of natural birth

- ✼ Research is showing that babies delivered naturally are more alert, exhibit greater interest in pre-breastfeeding behaviours and tend to spend longer suckling within the first 90 minutes.

- ✼ A drug-free, natural, vaginal birth reduces the possible risk of complications for both the mother and baby and reduces the need for obstetric interventions.

- ✼ Endorphins are secreted during a natural childbirth. These are endogenous opiates (like a mild morphine or heroin) that are secreted by the body to inhibit pain. Production of the hormone oxytocin increases until the moment of birth and creates a feeling of euphoria and increased receptiveness to the baby.

- ✼ These opiates have been discovered in both the umbilical cord and in the placenta. So they may also play a role as pain relief for the baby.

- ✼ With full feeling in an unmedicated body, the mother experiences all the birthing messages or the natural reflexes that occur during labor and birth. In natural childbirth, mothers generally are able to push better and faster because they can respond to the body's natural reflexes.

- ✼ Recovery after a natural childbirth can be faster and easier as the mother is able to move about and eat shortly after giving birth.

Labor and delivery pain

Your body design has evolved over countless thousands of years to give birth to your baby naturally. The pain of delivering your little one is real but is not the pain of, say, an accident that damages your body. In fact, labor pain is the opposite. It is the baby's way of constantly giving you messages about her progress now that she has decided to arrive. Pain is the signal that something quite beautiful, in fact absolutely awesome, is happening inside your body.

Preparing for pain

It is possible to prepare for pain so you can more readily accept and use it as a natural part of an unmedicated labor and birth.

- Firstly, don't avoid thinking about it whenever the thought pops into your mind. Begin to self-talk, telling yourself the positive things I mentioned above.
- Tell yourself that it is the baby's way of communicating lots of valuable data about her arrival. Remind yourself why you want a natural birth: perhaps, for example, so her little body wouldn't be affected by drugs.
- Relax into the pain rather than fighting against it—in other words, work to let go anxiety and fear which only makes you tense and, in turn, increase the level of pain. (Again, read the mother-stories of encouragement.)
- Use your meditation to do this. Apply your skills of deeply letting go tension and slow breathing for calmness. Review the section on meditation and pain relief before you go to the birthing place.

Medicated birth

Although natural birth is nature's way, there may be circumstances in which you are grateful that you can obtain pain relief when it is chosen or needed. It can be, for example, the most wonderful resource if labor has been intense for an overly long period or if the body is becoming too tense and anxious during contractions (but meditation does that too).

The main pain reliever available is an epidural, which partly numbs the expectant mother from about the waist down. I have observed the relief this provides to women whose pain goes 'over the edge' if the baby is just not cooperating. The upside is the argument that the birth is more enjoyable as there is virtually no pain. The downside is that it can prolong labor by lengthening the time needed for pushing.

Epidurals may also increase the possible need for further intervention to assist birth as the body is not able to work with its reflexes. There is an increased risk of baby damage from such intervention. (I carry head indents and bumps from a forceps birth.)

The decision to medicate—agreeing to intervention

Some say that, if the decision is made for pain relief rather than being a medical imperative, this may be against your long-held wish for a natural birth. Later you may have some regrets that you weren't stronger. This, of course, is nonsense. Any woman giving birth in whatever manner has been magnificent and all have an equal opportunity to go on and be a wonderful mother.

But before making the final decision, seek the support of your partner and/or your birth-friend. They may encourage you with love and warmth to 'keep going for a little while'—which you almost certainly can. Also, question your caregiver on the benefits or disadvantages of any interventions you might undergo.

Quite simply, the more informed you and your partner are, the more likely the best decisions will be made.

A cesarean—to have or not to have

I liked the idea of knowing what day and time my baby would arrive so I could schedule my parents to be here, a baby nurse, and furniture delivery.

—COURTNEY MIZEL GREEN[22]

Birth by cesarean section can be either elective (patient-planned in advance) or because it is deemed necessary for the wellbeing of the mother or child or both. Currently, there is considerable worldwide debate on the subject because more and more women are choosing to schedule a cesarean over a natural birth, thus removing the guesswork on the baby's arrival time for the same reason as Ms Green (who, by the way, finally chose a vaginal birth). To an increasing number of women, a cesarean is the way to remove uncertainty, fear and delivery pain: to have some control over the seemingly uncontrollable.

A planned cesarean does all of that and, in the recent decade, they have been so accepted that more than 30 percent of births in Australia are by this method, the highest rate in the OECD.[23] Interestingly, only about 4 percent are medically required as a safety intervention.

The bottom-line question has to be whether an elective cesarean offers any real advantage over a natural birth other than certainty of timing, greater efficiency in life planning and pain reduction. Supporters say that these are sufficient benefits and the American College of Obstetricians and Gynecologists (ACOG) adopted a position that stated that doctors may ethically perform an elective but medically unnecessary cesarean if it is 'in the best interest of the patient'.

That position has proved controversial, because any cesarean, in reality, is a major surgical procedure with all the attendant risks. There has been heated opposition to ACOG's views by other reputable women's healthcare organisations such as Lamaze International, the American College of Nurse-Midwives and the International Cesarean Network. The groups tend to agree that birth is a natural process and should be considered so unless there's a strong medical reason for surgical intervention.

A personal meditative thought is that, if an elective cesarean is chosen after a perfectly normal pregnancy, it also removes the baby's right to her decision of arriving when she knows better than anyone that she is perfectly ready to do so.

The decision, of course, is yours, to be mulled over with your partner and then passed on to all others concerned. As I've said before, your capacity as a caring mother can in no way be diminished by the method of delivery.

Cesarean and meditation

Having a planned cesarean is not a reason to let your meditation practice slip, even though you will not be using it for pain relief during delivery. Before and after the operation, your ability to let go tension and your slow, deep breathing will enable you to cope with any difficulties in a much more settled way.

Concluding thought on a birth plan

I suggest that you write down your own thoughts about the issues I've mentioned and even meditate upon them. This may well help you clarify your approach to the important event ahead. Whether you use it exactly as prepared, or not at all, doesn't really matter but it will almost certainly enable you to approach the final stages with a greater peacefulness of mind.

Driving to the birthplace—with meditation

This is where your months of practice begin to be mobilised as meditation in action. As soon as you go into labor, you can move into a mind-place where your various skills become your close companion for the days ahead. While packing the last few things, including your meditation items, you can begin slowing your breathing and deliberately letting go tension around your eyes. You'll soon find that you can remain perfectly calm during these early moments of rising excitement.

During the drive to the birthplace, keep your full mind-awareness on your breathing and letting go tension across your whole body.

It is the opportunity to remind yourself that you need to practice these essential elements of calmness as a priority now, all the way to holding the little one in your arms. Replace any apprehension with a smile and give her a loving rub. She's waiting to see you too.

Alison's story

Let go and trust

When I was pregnant with Arthur, I started a repeat course in meditation at the Meditation Sanctuary. It was around the middle of the pregnancy. I had recently taken a step up in my job as an architect and was managing a team working on a large building. During and after the course, I sat for meditation for half an hour each weekday morning. I remember feeling in control and calm throughout my work on that project despite the increasing lethargy and burden of my growing body.

My approach to the labor was to try not to have one!—not to have a 'labor plan' as is often encouraged – and to remind myself not to be afraid. The only plan I had was to go as far as I could without pain relief, hoping that 'as natural as possible' would be best for me and the baby. As it was my first baby and I didn't know what to expect, we chose to have the baby in a hospital so that, should intervention be needed, it was readily available.

In early labor, my husband and I had quite a few strolls around the block before evening arrived. When we arrived at the hospital, I was sufficiently dilated to be admitted. It was around 11pm so I was still expecting quite a few hours of labor.

All this time I focused on breathing through the contractions and relaxing between them. For this relaxation I used the letting go techniques that Brahm teaches and came to have a little routine. I would say, 'Relax eyes, relax shoulders, relax arms, relax thighs' as many times as I could before the next contraction started. I felt in control.

Our midwife suggested I try a hot shower where I ended up staying for three hours. During this time the midwife suggested I take the gas in the shower so I took that for a while. In retrospect, I can see now I lost my relaxation reminder when I started on the gas. Although breathing the gas gave me something else to focus on, I now wonder if this change was a turning point.

At some stage I realized I wasn't sure if I was having contractions— they had slowed to almost nothing. By 6am there had been little progress to the labor over the last couple of hours. And it was staff change-over time for the midwives. The midwife who had been with us for part of the night announced on her departure that I needed syntocinon to move the labor on again and should therefore have an epidural as I was tired.

We were very lucky that the attitude of our new midwife was more aligned with our own.

He encouraged me to rest but when the contractions did not start again, he suggested the syntocinon drip but starting with a low dose. He didn't mention the epidural. My husband says at one point the doctor came to the door saying he'd heard an epidural was needed and the midwife didn't let him past the curtain!

Although my memory is sketchy, I can say how, from this point, my meditation and yoga practice were of enormous benefit. I let go. Entirely. I didn't have any fear. I didn't need to tell myself not to—it was just not there! I let my body do its work. I simply followed the directions of the midwife and did not fight the pain. I am quite sure this ability to let go and have trust was much born out of practicing meditation and yoga.

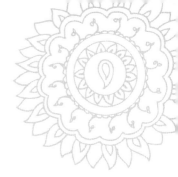

CHAPTER FOURTEEN

Meditation for labor and delivery

In this chapter, I briefly describe the three phases of labor but, unlike the trimester chapters, I enclose the meditation practices *within* the various development phases of the labor so you will need to have read, practiced and understood them. Do refer to Part One for a refresher at any time. My suggestions are only guidelines because you now know the effects of the Three Essences and can apply whichever one you think appropriate to optimise the benefit needed at any time.

If this is your first baby, your labor may last around 10 to 12 hours—sometimes longer. If you have previously experienced a natural birth, the average time may be around eight hours, but it is not uncommon to be less—or more. In the final analysis, your little one will decide just how long she wants to take. The important thing is that you have the full array of meditative tools to help you through each of those hours.

Arriving—setting up the birthplace

It is an extraordinary fact that most animals, if their chosen birthplace is disturbed as they are settling for delivery, will suspend labor while they seek out a new location. Scientists are beginning to understand that the same may apply to our species as well—that a woman's labor may be longer and more difficult if she is stressed by rushing, and by excessive busyness and noise about her birthing place.

After arrival and while waiting for your room, there are many meditative tools that you can adopt. When not having to talk to someone, talk to your little one in your mind and stroke her by rubbing your belly. At the same time, you can pick out an object such as a picture on the wall and focus deeply on it, even just for a few moments, while letting go tension and slowing your breathing. Keep doing this even in little spells. Short-interval meditation can be powerfully effective, as you are probably already aware.

When you get to your room, you and your partner or birth-friend can set it up as you want it for calmness and meditation. Attend to the basics so that you don't have to worry about them as you progress. Perhaps ask for bright lights to be turned off or shaded. Then ensure your music and headset are nearby. Have your polished stone in hand or beside you the whole time. Place your meditation object where you can give it single-focused attention at will. How about having one lovely little flower in your favourite vase, just where you can see it smiling back at you?

As soon as you have settled into the birthing room, you can set a peaceful tone for the rest of the journey by listening to your music, gazing at your meditation object, perhaps lighting a stick of incense or dabbing on an aromatic fragrance. These activities alone will calm you significantly because they are comfortingly familiar to you.

The three phases of labor

The first phase

A good part of phase one will almost certainly be experienced at home. When your contractions have been maintaining a regular pattern and reasonably consistent length of time for an hour or so, you are in early labor, the first of the three phases.

You need to monitor the tempo of your early contractions and, from time to time, seek phone advice on your progress from your support team who will confirm the right time to head off, which is when the cervix is dilating towards about 4 centimetres of a possible 10 centimetres. You will certainly feel the contractions now as a tightening or a slightly painful squeezing but the pain is unlikely to be too severe.

Know that the baby is communicating with you and that contractions throughout your labor cause no damage. They are just the muscles going to work, stretching naturally to create an open pathway for the little one's final momentous journey.

Meditation in the early stage of the first phase

You are likely to feel excited and possibly a tinge of apprehension when you realize that 'this is it'. Labor has really begun and your baby is on her way after 10 months of living within you. This is a totally normal response, even though you have been practicing being calm for months and months.

- Along the way, I have guided you in the smiling meditation, a wonderful antidote to apprehension, in any situation.

- This is the one you can 'just do' whenever you feel a niggle of apprehension in the early stages. You can layer it over the top of your quiet breathing and tension-freeing practices.

- At the same time you can gently stroke your tummy and offer soothing humming to the baby. The humming soothes you too.

- When you are free of the hubbub, reinforce an environment of peacefulness with a longer meditation and then shorter ones until you reach the next phase of your labor when more specific practices can be employed.

You will find this early stage a wonderful time to meditate because there isn't a lot else to do. Labor involves quite a lot of waiting! In these meditations, the endevor is to actually reach as far as quieting the mind with your chosen technique and then letting go the technique as you know how so you can dwell in the serene space of genuine stillness. It can be a closed-eyes meditation or an open-eyes practice, focusing deeply on your treasured object.

- At some time before your contractions become too frequent or severe for long and deep meditations, I recommend you do one or two shorter open-eye meditations as a 'dry run' for using later when it is important to focus deeply on managing pain or apprehension.

- If you are finding it hard to settle into a deeper meditation in your new environment (perfectly understandable), don't worry about the Third Essence (quieting the mind) for a while.
- Just become absorbed in letting go tension and slowing your breathing, allowing the breathing to be as restfully deep as is comfortable. These two practices alone will bring you the calmness you have already experienced.

The active phase

The early phase ends when your contractions gradually become more frequent, longer and stronger and the cervix continues to open. The active phase is in progress.

Contractions will become increasingly intense but slowly and gradually . . . in such a way that your body familiarises itself with the progress. It can be reasonably painful at the peak of the contraction. Over the next hours, you will move through the active phase where your cervix will dilate to around 8 centimetres.

The final stage of phase one is called the transition, where the cervix dilates to about 10 centimetres. It is birth-ready then and so is the baby. Contractions in this transition period can be very intense, lasting a minute or more and coming about every three minutes.

The break between contractions is rarely considered as a time of great value—just a time of understandable relief when the pain has eased for a while. But the time between contractions becomes very important for you because, knowing meditation, you can use this time to prepare for your next contraction.

Meditation in the active and transition phases

Dr René Frydman[24] says that 'it is not called labor for nothing'. It is throughout this phase, however, that you really can make your labor easier than it might otherwise be. Your practiced skills can now be switched to 'full on'.

The smiling meditation is no longer sufficient. I suggest the following steps as a kind of blueprint, but there is no absolute rule on which practice to use and when. Only you can know which one to pull out and use. Ask your partner or birth-friend to encourage you with suggestions if or when you begin to 'lose it' for a little while.

Letting go tension between contractions

* When a contraction has completed, try not to get into a long discussion or indeed, any discussion.

* There is always a minimum of some minutes before the next one arrives so, as soon as the last contraction has eased, move to a total 'chocolate melting', whole-body letting go.

* Keep your mind-awareness in your body. Let go thought of the last contraction by bringing yourself back to 'just this'. Say 'just this' aloud, even very loudly, if it helps bring your attention back to becoming absorbed in letting go tension.

- Deepen this focus by introducing your mantra humming to help you release more tension.
- Take your mind-awareness to your lower tummy area. Deliberately rest it by letting go as much tension as you can, inside and out.
- If you prefer, you can replace 'just this' and humming with an open-eyes meditation focusing on your object. (Many women have commented that they find this a better way because there is something tangible outside them to take attention away from the pain.)

Tension during contractions

Letting go tension can be profoundly effective in easing the pain of labor because you are working on calming the body which, as you know, paves the way for a calm mind. It is a wonderful way of easing apprehension while waiting for the next contraction. This actually works. Have another glance at Vanessa's story in the Prelude on page 14.

- When contractions become severe during the transition phase, focus single-pointedly on the lower tummy, just as you practiced in your early meditations.
- Endevor to let go as much tension there as you can while keeping the rest of your body as tension free as possible.
- Grip and squeeze the stone as pain becomes more intense.
- Work hard on keeping your mind on the job. Others will be encouraging you – but encourage yourself too. Talk

to yourself: 'I can do this' . . . 'I will see you in a little while', and so on.

Breathing between contractions

❀ Between contractions, as you are letting go tension, slow down your breathing until it is gentle again.

❀ Count both in- and out-breaths if you need to in order to slow them down. The counting becomes your point of focus.

❀ When your breathing has slowed, endevor to breathe as deeply as you comfortably can. With the baby having moved down, you will find that this can be a little deeper than your recent 'normal'.

❀ Keep bringing your mind back to 'just this' calming, rhythmic breathing. Remember, the more tension-free and calm you are, the less intense the pain you may experience.

Breathing during contractions

❀ In the early phases, you can maintain the method above, but there will come a time, as contractions become more severe, when slow, deep breathing is just not helping you through.

❀ Endevor to avoid rapid panting for air. Panting takes energy, all of which you need to reserve for pushing soon.

❀ It is better to breathe more slowly but use the high-oxygen intake method of dynamic breathing. Remember, dynamic breathing is breathing into your whole lungs and breathing out forcefully from your whole lungs at the same time—through pursed lips if that helps. Remember, this only uses approximately one-third of the energy-sapping effort required for panting and enables you to remain much calmer under duress.

The second phase

The second phase begins when the cervix is fully dilated. This is the 'pushing phase'– the final descent and birth of your little one. This phase can last from a few minutes to a few hours. In this phase, your baby's head keeps moving down with each push and then it crowns. This means that the top of the baby's head is visible. The midwife may show you in a mirror or guide you to feel for yourself, both wonderfully encouraging. In some places, particularly in Europe, you might be invited, after the shoulders have emerged, to reach down and deliver her yourself.

During the pushing stage, you are likely to be coached as to just when to push. You may be asked to stop after the head has emerged so the doctor can check that the neck is free from the umbilical cord. Then you will need to push again. Her head will turn, as the shoulders rotate into position for their exit and then . . . the rest follows!

Meditation during the second phase

Particularly in the final stages, you may find your practiced ability to focus on 'just this' more valuable than at just about any other time. It is time to go to work, directing your saved-up energy in a focused way for pushing to deliver your baby. There may be a number of pushes, from two or three to quite some more. There will be a period of rest between pushes.

During pushing

These are the long seconds of maximum effort.

* Take a very deep breath.

* With a real intensity of will, take your entire mind-focus to 'just pushing hard'.

* If you need more breath during a push, fish-mouth out and do dynamic breathing in again a couple of times and hold your breath.

* Re-focus and keep pushing until the kind helper tells you to stop for a bit. Keep holding that stone!

Letting go tension between pushes

* In the period of relative quietness between pushes, resume dynamic breathing for a short while to get back sufficient oxygen.

- Then as soon as you can, begin calming down again by gradually slowing your breathing.
- As best you can, move quickly to letting go tension in the whole body. This will give you so much more energy for the next push than lying/sitting there panting hard and waiting apprehensively for the next one. Utilize the time to renew yourself. Even just a little is of tremendous value.

At the moment of delivery and seeing her little face, you will have a range of emotions flood over you like a fresh waterfall. You may be exhausted but the hormones kick in and you will feel euphoric, wonderment, relief that it is over, a sudden rush of love for your partner and just about everybody and then probably, a complete sense of awe when you first reach for your baby.

The journey is over . . . and has just begun.

The third phase
The cord has been cut, possibly by your partner. Effectively, at the moment of birth, the third phase has begun. This involves a resumption of relatively mild contractions that soon deliver the placenta. In the excitement of holding their baby, some new mothers barely notice these contractions. The birth is then complete.

The baby at birth
She has just spent months tucked into a little ball in your uterus, so

she is going to look a little scrunched up for a while, her little arms and legs not extended and she may actually be bow-legged. By six months, all this corrects itself. No matter what, she will be the most beautiful thing you have ever seen.

Selena's story

Staying calm is the key

My baby, Max, was due on 14 October 2009. A few weeks before he was due, I found out he was breech and I was devastated as the dream and image of the perfect natural birth began to slip away from me. However, I was determined to do whatever it took to turn this baby around. I used acupuncture and visualization, but nothing was happening. I ended up having a procedure at the hospital to turn him. It's called an external cephalic version.

This is when my meditation practice first came into play. Little Max was so comfortable and did not want to move. It took all the strength of a male doctor to turn him and all of mine to block out the pain. There was only a 30 percent chance of turning but, amazingly, he did. Success! The doctor was astonished that I was able to withstand the pain with no screaming or crying. I just blocked it out and focused on the natural birth I was going to have.

I was so happy that I could then relax a little and enjoy the last weeks of being pregnant. After the procedure, I began to have Braxton Hicks contractions that lasted until I was due . . . and then an extra 11 days!

I was booked in on Tuesday 28th to be induced. On the Friday before, I went in for a check-up to see if I was close to going into labor. The doctor said not at all and that he didn't think it would happen on its own. I really didn't want to be induced.

The next day I woke at 3am in pain. I was in labor—it was happening! I spent the day walking around and doing what I could to help my baby arrive. I was so calm, but excited.

After laboring at home until 11pm on the Saturday night, we went to the hospital and were told it was close. I walked around as much as I could and took hot showers. At 3:30am, I told the midwife I had an urge to push so this was it. I was still fine, in pain, but managing it. I began to push and the pain was not that bad. It took 90 minutes and at 5am, Max was born . . . and I did it all medication free!

I believe I was fine because I believed I would be. With meditation, I stayed calm during my contractions and there was only one point where I felt I was losing control . . . pretty good, I think, considering the 26 hours of pain added to a complete lack of sleep.

I found it so important to have the practice of meditation available to me . . . especially to the point where you can practice in any place with any distractions, not just in a quiet room with candles. Staying calm is the key. Ironically, the worst pain I felt was when I momentarily felt a loss of control. Fear causes more pain than anything.

I did it all on my own and feel so proud and always think of the whole experience in a positive way. I was so glad to have my natural hormones doing their job.

What a rush when they gave me my baby, Max! I was then able to hold him on my chest for an hour . . . a really important bonding time.

CHAPTER FIFTEEN

Meditation: bonding and 'the blues'

The welcome must be thoughtful and respectful. We put a newborn on its mother's belly for instance, because the baby likes it, not only the mother. We know why it likes it. The baby finds some prenatal marks there, the scent of its mother, her body warmth, her voice, all sorts of marks very reassuring to the baby's sense of self.

– Dr Myriam Szeje[25]

The medical care can wait . . . it's very important that the baby feels welcome (because) it can affect the way the baby approaches life. We don't know how much the baby understands our words but we assume it deciphers the intentions beyond the

words . . .(but) any emotion on the mother's part clearly
affects the baby.

– DR MARIE-CLAIRE BUSNEL[26]

Make sure they don't take your baby away to weigh or clean
straight after the delivery. The baby should be given straight to
the mother with skin-to-skin contact. I was lucky enough to have
this experience and they did not take Max away to be weighed
for over an hour. I never had a problem with Max attaching or
bonding. The father should also take the baby and have skin-to-
skin contact.

– SELENA, MOTHER AND MEDITATOR

From the womb to the world: the first hour

Doctors and psychologists worldwide are now beating the drums loudly about the management of the baby's first moments, minutes and hours after the birth. Their discoveries, knowledge and opinions are today being reinforced increasingly by the true experts—mothers, who are providing wise commentary on the value of keeping the baby with them, skin-to-skin, from the moment the cord is cut for at least an hour, or more if they wish.

What a change from the old days, when children were whisked away virtually immediately for checking, weighing, washing and injecting. With my youngest son, I objected and was reluctantly given permission to carry him and be with him during the above procedures. That was just 20 years ago.

In other parts of the world, our recent western-world 'discoveries' of immediate mother-comforting upon birth have been known for countless centuries and by the animal kingdom from the beginning of their existence. In many species of chimpanzees, for example, the baby maintains skin-to-skin contact, without a single separation, for a number of months. They then stay within direct eye-contact range for the next seven years! I presume their little ones all grow up to be very good and psychologically secure chimps. There is a lesson there somewhere.

One example of a similar approach in the human species is the Latino tradition of *cuarentena*—the quarantine. The mother spends 40 days resting with the newborn after delivery and her only concern is caring for the baby. The wider family maintains the house, cooks all the meals and watches over any other children.

What science is now able to explain is that the first three months of a baby's life, from the second she is born, are critical. What happens to her in this delicate window of time can influence and shape the kind of person she turns out to be for the rest of her life.

Researchers' work is showing that, at the moment of birth, only about a quarter of a baby's brain is formed. The remaining 75 percent yet to be developed is mainly the 'wiring' or the connections between the cells . . . most of which develop in the first 18 months or so, with the whole growth project finished by about the age of seven.

In his brilliant, best-selling book, *Baby on Board*,[27] eminent Sydney neonatal pediatrician, Dr Howard Chilton, wrote:

This new (neurological) information confirms what the developmental psychologists have been saying for 30 years: how babies are managed during the time when they are making these connections is really important for their long-term mental health. For years it was assumed that the way individuals made these connections was purely genetic and was not much influenced by the world around them. We now know that that view was incorrect. It seems the way babies are brought up—their experiences, relationships and surroundings—profoundly change the way their brains make these linkages.

The neurobiologists call this *plasticity* (which makes the developing brain so susceptible to parents' attitudes and behaviour), and that is the reason for full-on attention to an immediate, loving, bonding start with all newborns.

Quite simply, the evidence from modern scientists of all relevant fields is that the behaviour and attitude shown to a baby from the first moment of its external life (and even in the womb) is the beginning of shaping that little person's whole being.

Meditation—the first hours and days

You might think that you are not going to have a moment to yourself for meditation in those first hours and days—and probably not for a long time. Well that's not quite true. From the moment your baby is handed to you, there is your beautiful 'object' on whom to focus attention.

So, here are a few possibilities for simple practice, but potentially so meaningful in setting her on a momentous life-path shaped by a brain 'wired' with love, warmth, comfort and security. You can use these practices during feeding time or whenever you need to soothe her and, indeed, yourself.

* When you put her to the breast, use her face as your point of focus. She can see you at that close distance.
* Soften your expression as in the smiling meditation.
* For a little while take you awareness back into your body, letting go tension from around your eyes and then from the rest of your body. She will feel this immediately.
* Slow your breathing. She will feel the quieting effect of that too.
* Move your awareness to her face and quieten your mind to 'just this'—gazing lovingly.

* You may want to hum gently, softly—something as simple as *OM* or *AUM*—because, if you have been doing this humming and chanting before she was born, she will recognise the sound instantly and feel the vibration of your chest through her little body – all so comfortingly familiar.
* Keep your 'other' object (flower in a vase perhaps) and your stone around. As you are the baby's comfort, so are these familiar objects quietly yours. Whenever you feel like it, or have times when you feel a bit lost, do a little open-eye meditation on the object while holding the stone.

There is a baby in the house—now what?

Giving birth is so often referred to as the 'happy event'. And indeed it is. You both have created new life and brought it into the world. But there the fairytale ends as the practicalities and responsibilities dawn upon you. Don't get me wrong. The nurturing of a child is mostly filled with feelings of love, spurred along by countless precious moments together that only you three experience.

In the early days and weeks, however, you are going to experience physical and emotional changes as significant as you did when you were in your early pregnancy. While endevoring to refine your ability to nurture and sustain a new life, you body begins to re-adapt to having this treasure on the outside rather than the inside. This is called the postpartum period and, during this biological transition, the baby in turn passes through a state of 'extrauterine adaptation'.

But she is almost unimaginably brilliant in adapting to the outside world. In just a few minutes, she has been transited, with the rudest of shocks, from being waited on hand and foot while floating peacefully in her own swimming pool, to actually having to breathe for herself, forage for food and then start seriously hard work in having to suck like there's no tomorrow.

These sudden changes for her and you are sufficiently daunting to make the physical and emotional health of you both a top priority.

Just for a moment, I want to look at an issue or two that can get in the way of truly and fully enjoying your little one's early life and how your skills in meditation might be put to work again. Some key difficulties can be bonding, postnatal depression (or postpartum blues) and the effects of simply forgetting to share and love each other as well as the baby.

Bonding

I have talked about post-birth bonding and it is true that many new mothers hit the ground running with arms full of mother-love for this long-awaited mite. That is the popular image, indeed, the expectation, of just how it should be. But the reality is that, for some very sound reasons, a love-bond with your baby can take a little longer to establish or the bond may be a little shaken when you have reached 'disc-full' exhaustion.

You have been through one of the most wearing and tiring experiences you are likely to have, even more draining if you layer on some anxiety and apprehension. In some instances, the new mom can be just too exhausted to express enthusiastic, unbounded love for the little creature in her arms. You may even think you are staring at a stranger. You are! But she is *your* little stranger and soon feelings of loving attachment will begin to grow and ripen, particularly if you have the intimacy of breastfeeding.

The most important thing is to let go any sense of guilt over any feelings about not 'falling instantly in love'. This is a new human in your life and, as you know, mature relationships with others blossom with nurturing—just like watering your flower garden.

Getting 'the blues'

Some new moms, however, may experience a feeling of ambivalence or even resentment lasting longer than a few days. If this is you and, after several weeks, symptoms begin to include anxiety, insomnia, detachment, tearfulness, moodiness, irritability, or even thoughts of harming either of you creep in occasionally, you are likely to be suffering postpartum depression. About 10 percent of new moms experience this kind of depression, which is due very much to the rapid and significant hormonal changes your poor, overtaxed body starts going through immediately after birth.

You have virtually no control over these biochemical changes, and experiencing depression in no way reflects on your capacity to be a great mother. The symptoms can make you quite unhappy, though, and you need to perceive that you aren't at top speed emotionally—and do something about it.

Meditation and postpartum blues

Many mothers have told me of their using meditation to ward off the blues. Interestingly, very few mothers who meditated seriously during their pregnancy experienced depression, and the several who did have symptoms commented that they weren't severe. I am not saying that meditation definitely will, or even will partially, prevent you becoming depressed, but there is strong evidence emerging that it can be of great value.

The mothers with whom I spent time on the subject, all agreed that recognising the feelings was the key to the effectiveness of the meditation. In other words, they were honest with themselves and, rather than let the feelings just well up and swamp them, they moved towards some preventative action.

This is a suggested approach to applying your meditation during a difficult time:

* Honesty first. Admit to yourself that you are feeling down.
* Then stop as soon as you possibly can for 10 or 15 minutes.
* Deliberately let go tension, focus deeply on your breathing and

stay with it for awhile, slowing and deepening as you know how.

- If possible, move to a meditation, letting go thoughts and then complete with a smiling meditation.
- Follow the meditation with self-chat ('this will all pass soon', 'if I can give birth, I can do anything', and so on), which can be comforting and beneficial.
- Practice mindfulness by constantly bringing yourself back to 'just this'. This is tremendously helpful in ensuring negative feelings don't take over to a point where you can't come back.

If symptoms can't be alleviated significantly by your meditation (and again, don't feel bad if you don't get on top of them this way), make an appointment with your medical professional who will help out. Also, don't keep it to yourself. Problems seem a little lighter if you have someone close with whom you can share your feelings.

But another key to not only surviving but perhaps getting through relatively unscathed is you clearly seeing and understanding some of the unnecessary obstacles that may be put in front of you. The task then is to apply meditation and your inner wisdom to build a solid, postpartum emotional base from which an optimum path of least resistance might be found for the first few months.

I suggest that the common factors in such a base for all mothers are awareness and understanding, then calmness, patience, perception and love, while again recognising that every mother will experience her motherhood journey in a unique way. As I said at the beginning, my aspiration for this book is to provide you with some natural tools not only to help enhance the experience of creating and nurturing new life but also to endure some of the difficulties you may face in the early months of your baby's life with a degree of equanimity.

Take great heart, though, that even if you are a deeply meditative mother-person, shedding some tears and getting your wheels bogged down in frustration is totally okay, in fact a very natural part of any optimum path.

Just don't forget to love yourself too.

A little chat to you both

It is so very easy to let go of each other a little or a lot while this baby takes the very large centre of a very small stage. Quite simply, dad can feel very left out and mom can feel downright unappreciated. But it doesn't take very much effort at all, just a little awareness, to build a lovely team spirit of personal inclusiveness.

You, the new mother, need to find simple ways to acknowledge that your partner remains an intrinsic, loving part of the ongoing creating and growing of this new life and helping to structure depth and dimension in her existence. Inclusiveness is critically important for you all. You don't have to do much. For example, you might tell your partner about little signs of progress or moments of interest that he missed. You might hand the baby to him, saying something like 'she needs a Daddy-cuddle' after you have fed her in the parental bed. Encourage him to put the baby on his bare chest and hum—watch and enjoy his pleasure in watching his baby fall asleep while he is holding her.

Perhaps of greatest importance are small gestures of genuine affection for your partner, such as a tender touch of his face or a gentle kiss placed on the top of his head as you walk by. Such little but intimate gestures can have a quite magnified effect of reassurance that he is not only included but truly loved as much as he always was.

You, the new father, have a similar responsibility in acknowledging this abrupt transformation in the family's structure.

To begin with, you have been an equal part in the creation of this beautiful newling and continue to be an equal part of her growth and development. In the earliest stages, although your holding, soothing, cuddling and talking to the baby is extremely important in creating your own bond with her, one of your major roles is deeply understanding that the key figure in nurturing the baby is her mother and that the majority of her attention, for awhile, will be directed towards your child.

Your role becomes much wider as you now support her by understanding her need to be with the child, telling her that she is doing a wonderful job, and physically helping out when asked or required. She needs to be reassured of your love for, and pride in, her. This can be exemplified by small loving gestures, even when she is busy or preoccupied with the baby. Gestures of loving warmth are so simple but so profoundly reassuring in really letting her know that the parental love-bond hasn't changed, but grown.

So just keep on loving each other—and show it, always. Therein lies a more complete happiness for everyone in this new family.

CHAPTER SIXTEEN

Meditation: reaching into your wisdom

Even before I left hospital, my head was reeling. I had 10 different opinions on just about everything to do with my baby, including breastfeeding.

– ALEXANDRA , MOTHER AND YOGA TEACHER,

In our modern, rapid-information society, there are many aspects of caring for a new baby in which current thinking and commentary offers such conflicting 'expert' opinions that the first-time mom is often becoming anxious, confused and even distressed.

Incredibly, much of the conflicting opinion centres around not the medical side of baby's basic health but the key natural aspects of the early nurturing of your little one: crying, comforting, feeding and sleeping.

For the meditating new mother, however, there is a way through the minefield of advice and opinion. In this chapter, I shall briefly discuss dealing with the bucket-loads of advice that new mothers face and offer a little further guidance so you may find a peaceful way through conflicting attitudes offered on just about everything. If you are then able to assess them with your meditative calmness and perception, you are much more likely to reach into the true understanding that the greatest wisdom on caring for your little one is inherent in both you and the baby, passed into your very genes through countless generations before you.

The modern erosion of confidence

We all know that nurturing a newling is never simple. In fact, the wise Dr Chilton suggests that you 'give up any thought of an ordered life for the first six months.' That there is conflicting thought, even at the professional level, on the management of the life of your own baby, still tends to astonish me because the females of the human race have managed to produce and raise their young reasonably successfully (or you and I wouldn't be here) for some 80,000 years and the forebears of our species for aeons before then.

It really is only a pinpoint in all of that time, the last hundred years or so, that mountains of opinions on 'big issues' (feeding, sleeping, crying and comforting) have been thrust before the new mom in so many different ways. And the debate on these core nurturing issues, just like the debate on natural childbirth, has been really heated.

Over these final chapters, I shall hopefully show you the ongoing value of meditation and throw a little light called 'common sense' on these issues so you might walk down the mom-path with more confidence, awareness and inner peacefulness.

Advice and data overload

The new mother is likely to experience a seeming bombardment of 'helpful' advice, whether asked for or not because, in this info-world, everyone is an expert. The days after birth are a time of increased vulnerability for you, weary still from giving birth and having the tiny one around-the-clock dependent upon you.

But this is a time, quite naturally, when advice is offered from a seemingly countless array of sources, many of them well-meaning, and perhaps others, in what I call the 'mother-industry', simply wishing to benefit from their ever-increasing services and wares.

Family outpourings, of course, are all an expression of love and good intentions. But along with the praise and adoration will come loads of absolutely unsought and, essentially, not-needed advice. You will soon find, however, that there are as many points of view as there are well-wishers. This can lead to inner conflict, which is beneficial to neither your nor your baby's wellbeing.

Know that the truly understanding family and friends will just love you, praise you and then get out of the way with no words of advice left ringing in your ears. Be warmly pleasant to all (the way of maintaining your inner peace) but make great effort to heed none of them . . . unless, of course, you specifically ask advice of a trusted wise one. Do everything the way you and your partner have chosen. You do not have to explain your approach to nurturing your child to anyone. Be comforted that, ultimately, you can't really go wrong because, as Dr Chilton says in *Baby on Board*, 'Luckily, human babies are as tough as old boots and hard to mismanage if they're loved.'

Today, there is also a mind-boggling amount of new knowledge readily available to the nurturing mother at the press of a computer button – mammoth quantities of data that would have made your mother's head spin and your grandmother snort in utter disbelief. For the new mother, however, the line between reassuring information and too much information can become blurred.

Constant checking to see if 'I am doing the right thing' can lead to moments of anxiety and apprehension. If you are a web-checker, ask trusted others for suggested sources of professionally accurate information. Seek out sites that offer wisdom based on scientific knowledge and not just opinion or points of view. Opinion has an agenda, wisdom doesn't. Wisdom is based on experience and provable knowledge.

You don't need to become a medical expert to bring up your baby beautifully—just a loving mother with your innate perception awake. When you find what you feel to be the right advice, meditate upon it for a little while. See if it fits with your natural instincts. Only proceed if it does, because deep down you really do know. If you get out of your depth for a bit, seek advice and help from your own trusted professional.

The glut of women's magazines, loaded with advertising and articles, as well as shelves of motherhood books dripping with advice and opinion, can be another source of understandable unease. The huge amounts of mixed messages can be enough to make your head reel with uncertainty at a time when there is just no need for doubts on the right way to nurture your baby.

My suggestion is that, whenever you are tempted to buy an advertised product or accept a media opinion on an issue or buy a book with a baby on the cover, first reach into your inner wisdom (it is always there) for advice and direction. Sit in meditation for a while, clear you mind and just let go. When you are ready, bring the issue before you and quietly look at it in mature contemplation. The answer will almost always be 'just there'.

It is a matter of having the courage to just listen to the innate wisdom of both you and your baby. Use your meditation to reach into your natural instincts and wisdom and also the wisdom to know when you need the advice of trusted others. Eventually, with ongoing practice of your meditation and mindfulness, you just know what is the right thing to do, buy or believe.

Ultimately, there is no right way—just your way, which, with loads of love and self-listening, will indeed be *the* right way, even if the way gets tough from time to time. If you create a little time whenever you can to practice, you will find that meditation is still your best friend and can keep bringing you little waves of gentle reassurance and calm confidence.

That 'tough-as-boots' little creature in your arms will always respond best to just being loved and treated with great care, compassion and warmth. I find it fascinating that this baby-rearing attitude I've just described is such ancient wisdom, yet in just the last decade or so is being touted as the latest thinking on bringing up baby. There's nothing new under the sun. Listen for the ancient wisdom within you.

CHAPTER SEVENTEEN

Meditation: enlightened guidance through the big issues

Feeding, sleeping, crying and comforting

These were the issues strenuously highlighted as the key difficulties experienced by so many new mothers to whom I have spoken or who have written to me in recent times. They began to stand out like beacons of particular relevance when many of those new moms reported dilemma, exhaustion, being 'at their wit's end', tearfulness, resentment, withdrawal, postpartum depression and, occasionally, being 'driven to distraction' by not knowing what to do.

They are issues that have been so fiercely debated, so confusingly and repeatedly questioned, in recent decades. Despite new mothers' deep instincts and wisdom, there is no wonder that so many have difficulties in managing these core baby-caring activities in a natural way.

The reason why I wanted to provide a little commentary on the four key issues, however, is that so many new mothers indicated strongly that their ability to meditate was either a 'great help' or 'the only thing that seemed to work' in finding their way through lots of nonsense and back to a sensible, workable and comforting approach for both baby and parents.

If you have been practicing meditation, then you have an array of skills you can bring to bear on all of these issues. In addition, at 'key-issue time' there is the potential for the meditating person to move to at least a part-rescuing mode involving love, kindness and compassion. This may lead you to a much easier path for yourself through the early difficult months, and certainly have an effect on your baby, which will begin to mould a fine and lovely being for the rest of her life.

The meditative understanding of the great power of love, care and kindness is the masterly core of meditation and has been for countless centuries. Applied to the four major baby-raising difficulties, this ancient knowledge has just relatively recently become core science and baseline psychology in the medical and other professional advice now increasingly being offered worldwide to new mothers.

I would need another book to deal with the other thousand questions you will have, from wrapping to weight, dummies to drugs and from nipples to nappies. But there are experts out there on all such important questions. Use your wisdom to find them if needs be. They are people such as the aforementioned Dr Howard Chilton whose extensive qualifications should also include BCS (Uni S of L)—Bachelor of Common Sense issued by the University of the School of Life (which happens to be regarded by Zen monks as the highest qualification achievable).

So, in this chapter, I want to briefly look at the key issues, hopefully from a broad wisdom point of view that will encompass the understanding arising from meditation as well as the knowledge of scientific, psychological and neurological disciplines. In discussing the issues, I will suggest how meditation can be the way around what may seem to be, at times, insurmountable rocks on the new-motherhood path.

Breast or bottle or both?

That there is conflict at all on this subject still tends to astonish me because the females of the human race have only had breast milk available as the single source of initial nourishment for babies since forever.

It was in 1867 when Justus von Liebig developed the world's first commercial infant formula, Liebig's Soluble Food for Babies. His initial formula spawned a multi-billion dollar industry to a point where, in the 1960s and 1970s, general surveys suggest that only 21 percent of Australian babies were still being breastfed at the age of three months.

Since then, various government strategies slowly improved this figure, although there has been considerable tension between the marketing forces of big business and the protagonists for natural feeding; tension still filtering through the motherhood system, often leaving the bewildered new mother sitting right in the middle.

Dilemmas over feeding baby

Key concerns, cultivated exclusively in the modern era, are whether to:

* feed naturally or 'default to formula'
* permit the baby to suckle until she is literally full or for a scheduled period
* feed on demand (breast or formula), also according to a planned schedule
* if breastfed, how long should the young one (in months or years) have access to the breast.

Another dilemma was introduced into the issue with the last half-century push for women's rights. This movement focused attention on the plight of new mothers and their 'lack of freedom'. Emphasiz on rights seemed to culminate in a furore created in 2009 by an American columnist, Hanna Rosin, when she wrote a magazine article titled 'The Case against Breastfeeding' for *The Atlantic*. In it, she effectively said that there was no scientific evidence that 'breast was best' and stated that 'breastfeeding keeps women down'.

This article brought the issue to a public head, in which the immediate and worldwide response at last provided a clear, wisdom-based direction for new moms. The World Health Organization (WHO), UNICEF and the vast majority of medical professionals came out strongly with one voice: 'for health benefits and mother-baby bonding, breastfeeding is preferred.' Kate Mortensen of the Australian Breastfeeding Association,[27] observed that 'breastfeeding is the physiological standard for growth and development.' She also backed feeding on demand, stating in effect that feeding by strict routine is not supported by science.

For mothers capable of breastfeeding their babies, the leading national and international health agencies now recommend exclusive breastfeeding for the first six months of life. Although formula is acceptable when necessary, health agencies regard it as an imperfect approximation of breast milk because the exact chemical properties of breast milk are not fully understood. In *Baby on Board* Dr Chilton described the early use of cows'-milk formula as a nourishment source for infants as the 'largest uncontrolled experiment in the history of humans.'

There is a range of excellent reasons for mothers capable of breastfeeding their babies to do so:

⁕ Breast milk includes the mother's antibodies that help babies avoid or fight off infections.

⁕ A mother's milk changes in precise response to the feeding habits of her baby over time. It adjusts nutritionally to the infant's changing needs as it develops. Formula cannot do this.

* The bioactive ingredients in mother's milk are designed to continue building a perfect child. She had the perfect start in the womb and mother's milk is designed to maintain the perfect nutrition that was provided to her in the first 10 months before birth.

* While the baby is being fed by breast, not only is her need for food being fulfilled, but she continues to have the ultimate bonding experience—learning about love through skin-to-skin touching, smelling, hearing and seeing you. She is likely to grow up with a greater sense of security and psychological wellbeing.

* Women who breastfeed have a lower incidence of uterine and breast cancer.

If bottle feeding is necessary

Today, women who either cannot breastfeed their baby or choose not to have increasingly sophisticated formulas for their little one. Essentially, today's formulas endevor to duplicate the rich ingredients available to a new baby in mother's milk. If, for whatever reason, your baby needs to be introduced to formula earlier than you might wish, the most important thing is that you have no sense of guilt. Just do it and get on. An environment with tonnes of cuddles, laughter and love is actually the most important thing of all to a child's ongoing wellbeing.

Demand or scheduled feeding

At birth, the outer part of the baby-brain, the cerebrum, the neocortex or 'new brain', is totally undeveloped. There is no ability to learn by experience and no skill at thinking through issues. The centre of the brain, the brain stem, which runs the core functioning of the body (including the reflex to find food) is, however, in place. Babies also have a quite well-developed midbrain or mammalian brain. This enables them to produce strong raw emotions – love, security and attachment when they are held lovingly and, conversely, fear and distress if they feel hungry, vulnerable or alone.

Experts say that trying to train a yet-untrainable brain with any schedules can only result in fear and distress which, of course, has lifelong implications on emotional wellbeing. Accordingly, the science-wisdom is that there is no evidence for trying to train a new baby to drink to a schedule. So, in the early weeks, perhaps months, the advice is to let her feed as often as she wishes and for as long as she likes. Meditative wisdom suggests the same.

To comfort you a little, however, she quite quickly gets to know the difference between night and day and, sooner rather than later, will be sleeping longer at night and will gradually create her own primitive routine for when she wants a good feed and a cuddle.

If there is a need to introduce formula (you have to return to work, for example), the experts suggest that you mix it for as long as you can with some of your own expressed milk because of the antibodies and nutrients that cannot be replicated in formula. After six months, her immune system will have been sufficiently educated by yours to adapt to other food more readily.

Meditation and feeding

As I mentioned earlier, using your little one as part of your medi-tation, indeed, the object of it, increases the beauty and intimacy of your ever-deepening love for each other, as well as an inner calmness during and after the feeding for both of you.

So, the early emphasiz is on focused mindfulness but, naturally, if you do find time for some *zazen* with full-on mind-quieting, all the better. But, while your life is totally unscheduled, don't try to create a specific time for your sitting practice . . . let it happen when it will.

Sleeping

There are two aspects to this issue. The first is how to get a reluctant sleeper to sleep. The second is where should she sleep—in your bed, nearby you in your room or in her own room.

Getting her to sleep

In the very early days, once she is fed and tired from the effort, like most babies, she will almost certainly switch off and fall asleep, quite often on the breast. But about 15 percent of the new-baby population falls into the category of what is called 'supersensitive' babies – little ones who just don't want to go to sleep.

This issue can often be resolved with a little trial and error, a good dose of common sense and some meditative wisdom.

Firstly, remember from where she has just emerged. The womb is a very dull, warm place with muted light, continuous mother-body sounds, the rhythm of your heartbeat like a permanent calming mantra, and an overwhelming sense of uninterrupted calmness and security. Suddenly ejected from this blissful place, she finds herself in an unsettling environment of bright lights and sharp sounds. There are several steps you can try out to get her to sleep—partly by recreating the womb environment as best you can:

- Try 'topping her up'. The last few mouthfuls may be just what she needs to feel happy.
- Create dimmed light but not darkness (even in daytime).
- Never surround her with pure silence. That is deeply unfamiliar. So your voice singing or humming or very soft, monotonous music such as gentle chanting or sounds of the sea on the shore can all be effective.
- Pat her gently at about the same rate as your heartbeat with which she is so familiar.
- If she shows signs of getting upset, put her on your bare chest,

with her ear near your heart and hum quietly. This too can be quite magical. To this day, I remember my father doing it to me and then me to my little ones.

❋ A technique that I used was to gently stroke the area between the baby's eyes and just above the bridge of the nose. An automatic response is to close her eyes and after a little while, they tend to remain closed.

❋ Importantly, try to be completely calm. She picks up your vibes in a second and any impatience on your part can be sufficient to 'set her off'.

❋ If you hum or vocalise your mantra to settle her, let that be your time of a beautiful meditation as well.

Sleeping together (co-sleeping) or baby alone?

On this question, medical researchers, scientists, neurologists and this meditation teacher all tend to agree in principle. The consensus of the wise is that, as a minimum, the baby should be within the same four walls as her mother and ideally very close and in sensory contact for the first six months of her life . . . but not actually in the same bed.

Renowned authority on co-sleeping, Dr James McKenna,[29] says bluntly, 'a baby sleeping separately from its mother is a baby in crisis.' In terms of sleeping with your baby, McKenna asks the question, 'Is it safe *not* to sleep with your baby?'

The suggested ideal is to have your baby's bed snug against your side of the parental bed so you can place a comforting hand on her in a split second or lift her to you when there is a 'need for feed'. Your immediate presence reduces anxiety and is of immense psychological and emotional comfort for you both. Having had constant physical contact with your little one for the past 10 months, it is also a natural instinct to keep the newborn close, day and night. Another co-sleeping option is that you have a bed next to her cot in her room.

Co-sleeping is supported by SIDS and Kids whose figures show a 50 percent less chance of a little one dying of Sudden Infant Death Syndrome if the baby is next to the mother on a separate surface (cot by the bed). A safe sleeping program in Australia has cut SIDS deaths by 85 percent in the last 20 years.

The counter-argument to co-sleeping is that bringing baby into your bedroom will make it dependent and, in the long term, create a rod for your own back. There is no scientific evidence for this and I refer you back to my comments on trying to train a yet-untrainable brain.

How to introduce sleeping independence

When the time is right, you can gradually develop the baby's sleep-time independence by initially placing her in a cot in her room for daytime sleeps. Make it womb-like (dim and boring). In the beginning, leave her for just a few seconds at a time before returning to rest your hand on her gently while murmuring quietly.

Increase the time of separation slowly by a minute or so every few days, although always responding and calming her if she becomes upset. In this way, the baby gradually is reassured that you are there and she is not alone.

In longer separations, another little ploy is to hum quietly in the next room before returning to lay a hand on her so she gradually loses the clear distinction between you being present right there or somewhere close. When the baby is a little older and aware that her 'home-base' (you) is around during her daytime sleeps, perhaps between, say, four and six months, you can ever-so-gradually effect the same result at night by following a similar procedure.

Begin by moving her bed a little further from you in very small increments. Eventually, of course, she will be sleeping longer and longer during the night and you will simply know the right time when she is safely ready to sleep in her own room—although you will find yourself wisely checking on her quite frequently for some time.

Comforting and crying

The settling of a crying infant has become one of the most contentious mothering issues, with many books written on the subject. It is one that can cause genuine family upset and requires some loving understanding and, again, some wise common sense to navigate through to quieter waters.

All babies cry for the simple reason that making a noise is their only way to communicate. Each time they cry, they are sending you a message to 'come to me now and fix my problem'. The responsibility of both parents is to learn to understand why she is crying and how to respond.

The baby-messages in crying

Your little one will cry for an array of different reasons. Many cries are usually just a quick response to an immediate, harmless stimulus. For example, she may have brief restlessness in her sleep and whimper-cry for just a few seconds or because she has become unlatched from the nipple for a moment as she is just starting to feed. Such crying responses are normal and usually resolved by the baby herself in a few seconds.

But all other cries are important. They can be an intense primal expression of anguish, the only response a baby can have when she feels the slightest threat to her very survival. In her early months, such cries are saying, 'I really am in need.' The primal cry is a serious call for your intervention and help because her outer brain is not sufficiently developed yet to manage overcoming issues by herself.

In the newborn, the primal cry can have several causes. The main one, of course, is hunger, resolved by feeding. The second is physical discomfort including pain, which can be treated according to the problem. The third is weariness, solved by lulling her to sleep. The fourth is fear.

Her main fear is of being abandoned (a total threat to her

survival), which is totally understandable because she has already experienced such a huge initial shock to her little system in leaving 'home'. Her first primal memory of abandonment can be substantially diminished by your immediate and loving tenderness at birth. However, being unexpectedly left alone, particularly in silence, is the baby's worst nightmare and will certainly cause a fearful crying for rescue.

Methods of comforting

Essentially there are three responses you can have to your newborn's crying. At one extreme, there is 'controlled crying' – just letting the baby continue to cry for a specific period of time. Then there is the middle ground that says crying is the way she gets her exercise, so let her go for a while because it is good for her. The other extreme, sometimes called 'attachment parenting', is soothing her as soon as she utters the first cry.

Controlled crying—for and against

Controlled crying is the most contentious of strategies in which the baby is left to cry until she learns to 'self-soothe'. The argument is that letting her cry is the antidote for her learning to manipulate you to jump to attention as soon as she whimpers and so develop a behaviour trend that could continue for years.

The issue of 'scheduled mothering' (including controlled crying) had quite some influence for several decades because letting the baby cry as advocated does put her to sleep—because she eventually collapses into sleep through physical exhaustion. Understandably, many worn-out mothers found peaceful release when the baby did fall asleep, not realising the potential damage to the child of controlled crying.

A number of mothers have told me that they soon gave up the practice because they felt 'trapped in a trend' that left them feeling 'pain, guilt and general distress'. They felt that ignoring a baby's crying through believing it was the right thing to do simply creates conflict in sensitive mothers which, unsurprisingly, accentuates the baby's distress.

Experts such as Dr Chilton describes books and advocates for controlled crying as a 'total disaster . . . being absolutely uninformed and unpleasant . . . and potentially destructive.'

Thankfully, supporters of controlled crying are becoming a dying breed as the results of recent scientific and neurobiological studies are being laser-beamed onto the issue and beginning to wipe out any legitimacy it may have held.

The formal argument against controlled crying is, firstly, the physiological damage caused by stress. In the first few months of life, the baby's outer brain is still developing as the emotional brain connections continue to be formed. If your baby is distraught, it releases exaggerated levels of the stress hormone cortisol. Neurologists are now showing that distressed and fearful babies may well become stressed adults who suffer such problems as anxiety and depression.

From a meditative point of view, I agree with Dr Chilton's con-clusion (among countless other experts) that it is not appropriate to walk away when a baby is distressed. I know that loving parents, listening to their instincts and inner wisdom, find it impossible to leave a crying child, no matter what an outside 'expert' may tell them is the 'right thing to do'.

Crying as good exercise?

There is an adage that 'crying is good for a baby; it strengthens her lungs.' There is no evidence for this. A baby's lungs continue to naturally develop over the first six months, just the way the rest of her complex little body has already matured naturally. The completed primitive brain has the progress of this entire new being under expert management as long as she gets sufficient nourishment and is not emotionally damaged.

Soothing the tears on demand (attachment parenting)

The final alternative response to an upset baby is soothing on demand. The argument against this is probably best summed up by the feminist author Erica Jong[30] who suggested that being 'ever-present' for our children became a parental 'prison' and was the 'ultimate bondage for women'.

It certainly may be for awhile, but the choice to have a baby seems to imply a profound and ready willingness to give your progeny every opportunity to grow up with a healthy body, mind and attitude. Certainly, the mature parent wants to develop the baby's independence, but the way to do this is to guide her there gradually, while underpinning her sense of security and developing her confidence, which can be so easily shattered by being left alone, crying for help.

In Zen meditation, we understand that, at the very core of every human, there lies a deep well of love, kindness, compassion and concern for the welfare of others. A crying or unsettled baby drills a well straight into these qualities, which innately compels your natural response to soothe.

The key ways of comforting

In summary, experts worldwide are saying quite simply, but very loudly, that you cannot cuddle, comfort, caress or kiss your baby too much. So do it whenever she asks for such loving attention and then, do it more often.

There are many ways to comfort a little one. Most of them are similar to getting her to sleep.

- Check that there is no overt cause of discomfort such as a wet or soiled nappy.
- Try feeding her. The act of suckling itself is called a 'stress regulator'. Suckling releases those nice hormonal opiates, which make her feel better.

- When she's upset, pick her up and cuddle her against your chest, so she can hear your heartbeat. Just that familiar, consistent rhythm is beautifully lulling for a tiny one and, indeed, is effective for children up to three and four years of age when they are discomforted and unhappy.

- In the Meditation Sanctuary, we often play gentle repetitive chants, or practice humming, rhythmically and softly to quieten the body, breathing and mind. Even to a stressed adult, this can be compellingly calming. Try that. The most comforting sound, of course, is your own voice. So, to ease fear-crying, just keep talking normally, but soothingly and gently.

- Be there and around her as she is developing. Through deep meditation, I have been able to recall aspects of my own very early life with great clarity. A standout memory when I was about four months old was of my being in some kind of low bassinette, but under the kitchen table! I can recall being fascinated by the markings on the underside of the table, while seeing the top of a tree swing in the morning sun outside the kitchen window. I distinctly recall a sense of comfort in being able to see just my mother's legs while she did the washing up to the familiar sounds of the radio pips and gongs and music ... all remembered with a sense of delight. Years later, she told me this was all true—she used to put me under the table 'so she didn't step on me'. This was a wonderful thing as she was not a small woman! The main point, though, is that she was 'just there' for me.

- If your baby is fed and fresh but just unsettled, walking with her in your arms is good. The lulling rhythm of meditative walking and breathing, walking and breathing, slowly and gracefully, can be quite magical.

- I know it's hard when you are on-your-knees exhausted, but try and be a soothing, calm person in your manner, movement and speech. Not only does it calm the baby but it makes your day so much better when you deliberately let go agitation as often as you can.

Continued distress

Deep down, all mothers really do understand the meaning of their baby's crying out for them. You do too and, as your confidence blossoms, you will increasingly be able to comfort her in a meaningful and loving way. But there can be occasions when the baby is telling you she is in really serious trouble, not just hungry or feeling abandoned. If her crying ever sounds like shrieking or genuinely pained and it continues despite your best efforts at comforting, it is time to visit the doctor.

Meditation and comforting

The very way you respond to your baby's need for comfort is a reflection of your loving kindness. In other words, responding to her with your innate and natural wisdom in a compassionate way is a pure practice of authentic meditation. Compassionate loving is putting your meditation to work in the way it is meant to be used.

You now have the techniques of meditation and mindfulness available to you always. You may be getting little time to yourself but when you do get a moment (such as during her day sleep), try to sit meditatively for a few minutes for a refreshing 'top up'.

In the more difficult early times with your precious child, meditation can be your very best friend.

Sandra's story

The power of meditation to help cope with pain

I have long believed in the power of meditation to help one cope with pain. Several years ago after attending a three-day meditation retreat in

Cambodia, I suffered a deep burn to a leg during a motorcycle accident. The pain was excruciating, but there was no treatment available nearby, not even ice or water. I had two choices . . . panic or meditate. Having just finished an inspiring retreat, I chose the latter. I focused deeply on my breathing and on my experience of the pain itself. To my amazement I found that the pain just switched off . . . almost instantly. Despite the fact that I still have the scar, I had no pain from that burn at all except for the first few minutes.

Therefore, I had a great deal of confidence in the power of meditation to help me cope with childbirth. So I meditated regularly in my pregnant months and felt that this helped me, not only to connect deeply with my unborn child but also to view the approaching birth (my first) with calmness and confidence.

Like many expecting couples, my husband and I had hoped to have an all-natural birth to give our baby the best possible beginning to his life. Unfortunately, all did not go to plan. When I was one week overdue, my waters broke but the labor did not begin. Eventually, the hospital decided that it was necessary to induce the labor. That was a very disappointing moment for me because I knew the statistics . . . a large proportion of induced labors end up in a cesarean. That was completely the opposite of the birth we had envisaged. Nevertheless, because the health of our child was at risk we accepted that decision, but I have to admit, I cried for quite a while.

When the labor began, however, I was able to just focus on my breathing and to begin to go into that deep place of quiet within myself. There again I found the peace and strength that is always at the core of my being and which I am able to settle into when meditating. The intensity of an induced labor can be much stronger than that of a natural labor because the body does not have time to produce natural, pain-ameliorating hormones.

But by the time the pain became intense, I was feeling completely serene. I found that pain is like a vicious, snarling dog. Your initial instinct will be to run, but sometimes if you just decide to turn around and look the dog straight in the eye *it* will run away from *you* with its tail between its legs! At that point you realize that it really is a rather small and pitiful creature despite its pretensions to size. Pain is the same. When you really focus and go deeply into the pain itself, it suddenly seems a very small and insignificant thing—it may even vanish.

My labor was so calm that the midwives attending me slipped out of the room and called the other midwives to come and watch. At one point between contractions I raised my head and found that I had an audience of midwives sitting quietly and watching. The other midwives who were not attending me came to just sit in the room where I was giving birth whenever they were not busy. They said that this was 'the beautiful room'.

Doctors kept coming by to offer me pain relief. They told me that there was no need to 'martyr' myself to the pain. They told me that it was all well and good to want a natural birth, but when things got difficult you should just take the pain relief. But I honestly didn't need it. The pain was there, but it was never something that was beyond my coping. Nevertheless, the inevitable happened and when the baby's heart rate began to drop from the intensity of the labor, a cesarean was scheduled.

My beautiful Alejandro was born healthy and happy despite all these dramas. Once again meditation helped me through those first few days in the hospital. My husband and I could hear babies screaming all over the hospital while our room was again peaceful and serene. The nurses kept putting their heads in the door to ask if we were alright, because everything was so much more quiet than normal. Again, midwives started escaping to our room whenever they could to enjoy the quiet.

Eventually we got home from the hospital and mothering began in earnest. The initial bliss of holding my beautiful newborn in my arms at last wore off. I found to my surprise that actually being a mother has been much more challenging than childbirth ever was. That was the easy part if you ask me. There has never been a challenge to my equilibrium or to my whole sense of self as great as motherhood. It's not easy to stay sane when you are sleep deprived and barely have a moment to think, let alone eat or have a shower. Where was the resourceful, efficient businesswoman that I used to be?

But still, the ability to go inside that quiet space within me has helped me to survive. There are times when a small baby just cries and cries and there seems nothing you can do to help them. At those times it is easy to think, 'my life is over', 'I should never have become a mother', 'will I ever sleep again?' But I tried to just hold him through those difficult times and to stay present and connect with him in his distress.

I can honestly say that I think the techniques that I have learned through meditation have saved my sanity. I am still at the beginning of my journey as a mother and have no doubt that there are more challenges and pains ahead. But one 'tool' I will be able to pull out of my 'toolbox' in any situation is meditation. It's not going to make me a perfect mom, but I will certainly learn a lot along the way.

'I like lizards': a meditative conclusion

Not so long ago, I gave a speech on the benefits of Zen meditation at a large annual event for a national organisation on health and wellbeing. I was the first speaker and was scheduled for the 9am time slot, too early for both speaker and audience, I suspect. Despite the ungodly hour, there was a large crowd, many still clutching coffee cups and wiping the sleep from their eyes. I was to speak for some 40 minutes, followed by question time.

As I prepared myself and then looked out at the blur of seemingly disinterested faces, I had a sinking feeling that getting their attention so early in the day was going to be a 'big ask'. Although the chairman had been very gracious in his introduction of me, I still felt the audience seemed to be settling in resignedly for a long and boring speech.

My first words were, 'I like lizards.' The change in the audience was quite electric. Heads lifted and I could see them wondering what on earth was this guy on about, particularly as I spent the next two or so minutes talking about the absolute delight I get in watching backyard lizards – those little skinks hilariously playing hide-and-seek between their daily duties of making their homes under the avocado leaves, finding food, bringing up their families while all the time being mindfully alert for any bird-enemies.

I finished my chat on these little skink entertainers in my backyard by saying 'These little lizards are just so busy . . . so very busy . . . being lizards!' My point was that they are living naturally and in perfect harmony with their environment.

I went on to say that 'People, like lizards, are so busy—except for one critical difference. People are so very busy *not* being natural humans in glorious harmony with their existence but spending their busyness trying to be *anything but* human.'

By this time, I think the audience had well and truly woken up so I added, 'It is fair to say that the human species, of all the species on the planet, is the one species that has lost all sense of natural harmony with its environment, the universal cradle which provides life.'

The point of my relating this story here is that every mother, including you, dear woman, is a universal cradle who provides life. Mothers provide in their wombs the perfect environment for nurturing their young. Deep within each mother is a profound, inherent knowledge and wisdom, passed to each of you through the genes of time, of being able to create a metaphorical 'nest under the avocado leaves' for your young one after birth and to provide so exquisitely and naturally for its 'perfectly harmonious existence'.

Science in recent times and across many wonderful disciplines and technologies has indeed given us great knowledge of, and consistent answers to, the inevitable dilemmas of delivering a baby to the world and raising it responsibly. Our knowledge of everything, from the hormones that 'help us fall in love' to procreation, conception, foetal development and the birth of a fully developed human, is increasingly intricate and awe-inspiring.

What really must be understood, though, is that from the moment of conception, and then particularly from the moment of birth, every young one begins a journey that is unique to her. In meditation, we understand that the totality of any person—their appearance, dress, manner, voice, way of behaving, attitudes, opinions and so on—is the sum of the billions of experiences they have had before they were born through to the lovely sunset they may have enjoyed last night, many years later . . . and every second of joy and suffering in between.

In recognising this uniqueness and in listening to the breadth of experiences of new moms, I have realized there is no 'magic bullet' that brings you the perfect pregnancy, perfect delivery and perfect way of positively influencing your baby's experiences. So, although we have mountainous knowledge on babies and all the textbook answers, there is not one recipe in existence that gives you a flawless, seamless passage through early motherhood. Similarly, there is not one piece of advice from well-meaning others, including me, that will give you the 'golden pass'.

So, precious mothers-to-be, if I may offer any advice, it is to have the courage to reach into, recognise and listen to your own wisdom first. All that you seek is within you, even the knowingness of those moments or times when you need to call upon another for help or guidance.

If you have been meditating, and indeed continue to meditate, I assure you that you will find it easier and easier to access this lovely inner spring of insight and understanding on 'just what to do'. You won't always get it right first up (remember you are a human, not a lizard), but that dear little one in your arms is extraordinarily resilient . . . and patient, and she will soon tell you that you might like to try something again or in a different way.

And all of this is made so much easier when you layer on your innate common sense. The naturalness of your watchful care and the cocooning of you both securely in mother-love will enable you all to happily enjoy your nest until the little one becomes a big one and is ready to leave.

So, a new life has been created—the evolution of humankind continues, the three of you playing your part in this beautiful universal play of existence. Moment by precious moment, celebrate this greatest of achievements.

May you all love each other beautifully and hold each other tenderly in your hearts for the rest of your lives. Bless you on this unique and wonderful journey together.

– Brahm

The End . . . and the Beginning

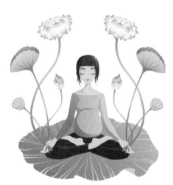

APPENDICES

LIST OF EXERCISES

First trimester

Second trimester

The third trimester

PHOTOGRAPHS

SOURCES AND REFERENCES

1   Geri Larkin *Stumbling Towards Enlightenment,* Celestial Arts, 2008.

2   *The Odyssey of Life* series, DVD, produced by Christin Gerin and Charles Gazelle (*see* Recommended reading and viewing).

3   Dr Sandra Cabot and Margaret Jasinska, *Infertility: The Hidden Cause,* WHAS Pty Ltd, 2010.

4   Professor Niels Skakkebaek, Department of Growth and Reproduction at Copenhagen University, first announced the decline in sperm counts in western men in 1992. He reviewed 61 international studies that had been undertaken between 1938 and 1992 involving more than 14,000 men. They found that the average sperm count had fallen from 113 million per millilitre in 1940 to 66 million in 1990. A survey of 1350 sperm donors in Paris found a decline in sperm counts by around 2 percent each year over the past 23 years, with younger men having the poorest quality semen. Subsequent studies have confirmed and strengthened Skakkebaek's findings. A male with a sperm count of less than 20 million per millilitre is considered to be infertile.

5   Dr Maurice Titran, pediatrician at Robaix Hospital, Robaix, France, founded the Early-Action Socio-Medical Centre in 1981. He was actively involved in the TV program *Le Bébé est une Personne* ('Babies are People Too'). He was in charge firstly, of Robaix's Early Childhood Program and then of the entire health program for several years. He headed the more recent national campaign in France about the ill effects of alcohol during pregnancy. From interview in *The Odyssey of Life* series.

6   Prenatal researcher, Benoist Schaal, National Centre for Scientific Research, Dijon, France. From interview in *The Odyssey of Life* series.

7   'The impact of lifestyle factors on reproductive performance in the general population and those undergoing infertility

treatment: a review', by G F Homan, M Davies and R Norman, Discipline of Obstetrics and Gynaecology, Research Centre for Reproductive Health, School of Pediatrics and Reproductive Health, Medical School, University of Adelaide, South Australia and the Adelaide Fertility Centre (Repromed, Dulwich) SA. Published in *Human Reproduction Update*, 2007, pp 1–15.

8   Interview, *Today* program, Channel MTN 9, Australia, 2011.

9   Dr Allen Morgan MD practicses fertility and reproductive endocrinology, obstetrics and gynecology in Lakewood and Ocean, New Jersey. From interview in *The Odyssey of Life* series.

10 Dr Elizabeth Blackburn, winner of 2009 Nobel Prize for Medicine, interview with Fran Kelly, ABC Radio, Australia, 6 October 2009.

11 Dr Jamie A Grifo MD PhD, Director of the Division of Reproductive Endocrinology at the NYU Medical Center in New York City.

12 Alice Domar PhD, Executive Director of The Domar Center for Mind/Body Health at Boston IVF, Assistant Professor of Obstetrics, Gynecology, and Reproductive Biology at Harvard Medical School and a senior staff psychologist at Beth Israel Deaconess Medical Center.

13 Dorothy Greenfeld, Clinical Professor of Obstetrics Gynaecology and Reproductive Sciences at the Yale Fertility Centre, Yale University, New Haven, Connecticut. From an interview in *The Odyssey of Life* series.

14 Dr Domar's study presented at the American Society for Reproductive Medicine's 65th Annual Meeting.

15 Dr Domar introduced the Mind/Body Program for Infertility at the BIDMC main campus in Boston, later moving it to Boston IVF in Waltham.

16 Francine Dauphin, renowned French activist and midwife. From an interview in *The Odyssey of Life* series.

17 Carolyn Granier-Deferre, developmental psychobiologist, Department of Neuropsychology, Paris Descartes University.

18 Carolyn Granier-Deferre, 'A melodic contour repeatedly experienced by human near-term fetuses elicits a profound cardiac reaction one month after birth', *PLoS ONE*, February 2012.

19 Aurelie Ribeiro, 'Near-term fetuses process temporal features of speech', *Developmental Sciences*, 2011, vol 14.

20 Anthony DeCasper, Professor Emeritus Psychology, University of North Carolina, 'Prenatal maternal speech influences newborn perception of speech and sound,' *Behavior and Development*, 1986, vol 9, pages 133–150.

21 Kelly Wider, commentator, Bellybelly.com.

22 Courtney Mizel Green, Los Angeles lawyer, Founding Director and Chairperson, Center for Empowered Living and Learning (The CELL). From her internet commentary.

23 OECD iLibrary and Australian National University Medical School, study, September 2009

24 Professor René Frydman MD is head of Gynaecology and Obstetrics at Antoine Béclère Hospital, Paris. From an interview.

25 Dr Myriam Szejer, child psychiatrist. Study published in *Prenatal and Perinatal Psychology*, 1996, vol 8; and 'Talking to Babies. Psychoanalysis on a Maternity Ward'.

26 Dr Marie-Claire Busnel, research pioneer into foetal perception, René Descartes University, Paris (*see* Recommended reading and viewing).

27 Dr Howard Chilton, *Baby on Board,* 2nd edition, Finch Publishing, Sydney, 2009.

28 Kate Mortensen, manager, Lactation Resource Centre, Australian Breastfeeding Association.

29 Professor James McKenna PhD, Edmund P Jaycs Chair in Anthropology, Notre Dame University, 'Sleep location and suffocation: how good is the evidence,' *Pediatrics*, 2000, 105(4).

30 Erica Jong, interview, *Wall Street Journal*, November 2010.

RESOURCES

Recommended reading and viewing

Dr Marie-Claire Busnel. *Le langage des bebes, savons-nous l'entendre,* Jacques Grancher, 1993.

Dr Sandra Cabot and Margaret Jasinska. *Infertility: The Hidden Cause,* WHAS Pty Ltd, 2010.

Dr Howard Chilton, *Baby on Board,* 2nd edition, Finch Publishing, Sydney, 2009.

J Hoffman, 'Hotmilk', www.todaysparent.com.

The Odyssey of Life series, DVD, Lagadère Entertainment France, www.VEA.com.au

Helpful websites

DONA International, www.dona.org

Babycenter, www.babycenter.com

Professor McKenna on infant sleeping, www.nd.edu/-alfac/mckenna

The Odyssey of Life, www.VEA.com.au (Subject ref. Health and Professional Development. Biology)

ABOUT THE AUTHOR

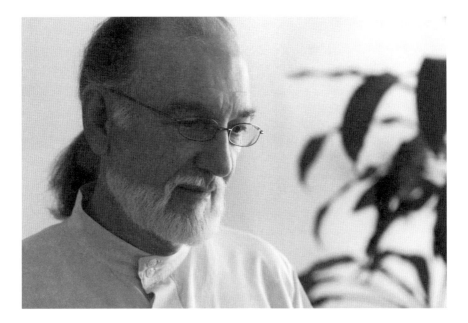

Yogi Brahmasamhara (Brahm) has practiced Authentic Meditation for about 40 years.

In the mid 1990s, he began teaching meditation and established the first Sanctuary in Leichhardt, Sydney, 15 years ago. Today, the Meditation Sanctuary attracts hundreds of students each year.

Brahm initially spent five years studying Integral Yoga with Indian Yogi, Misra Bashayandeh, who himself had been a student of the internationally renowned philosopher and Yoga Guru, Sri Aurobindo, at Pondicherry in India. He then refined his practice within the classic Soto-schu Zen tradition of meditation at the monastery of Japanese Zen monk, Suni Kaisan, on both a visiting and full-time basis over three years.

Born in Griffith, NSW, Australia, to farming parents, Brahm became a radio announcer at 16, before moving to Sydney to study theology. Meeting Bashayandeh gradually shifted his intended 'spiritual path' away from formal religion to exploring and studying the 'enthralling profundity' of meditation. Later, it was his Zen master, Suni Kaisan, who sent him into the world 'to experience life to prepare him' for teaching.

He did just that, working in various fields. He taught English language and literature at the University of New South Wales; produced some 30 documentaries on Australian artists; tasted the corporate world with a three-year stint in an international oil company and then established his own award-winning graphic design company. During that time, he co-authored a book on William Balmain (with Dr Peter Reynolds) and wrote poetry prolifically. He also spent much of his time competing around Australia as a motor racing driver – which he describes as 'an extremely meditative activity'. In the mid 1990s, he turned to teaching meditation as his teacher had foretold.

Brahm's first book, *Awakening: A Practical Guide to Zen Meditation*, was published in 2008.

MEDITATION SANCTUARY

yb@meditationsanctuary.com
brahmasamhara@optusnet.com.au
www.meditationsanctuary.com
Twitter: @zenwithbrahm
Facebook: www.facebook.com/ZenwithBrahm